Dr. Greg's Green Home Makeover

Your Family's Guide to Healthy, Sustainable Living

Gregory Charlop, MD

First Edition: 2023

Published by Dr. Greg LLC Atlanta, Georgia

For reprints or other inquiries, please contact Greg@visionaryremodels.com

ISBN: 979-8-9885229-0-4 (eBook)
ISBN: 979-8-9885229-1-1 (Paperback)

www.GregoryCharlopMD.com

Important Disclaimer

This book is for educational and entertainment purposes only. It is not a substitute for professional advice or services. By reading this book, you understand and agree that Gregory Charlop, MD, Dr. Greg LLC, its affiliates, and any contributors to this book are not liable for any damages arising out of the use, reference to, or reliance on any information contained within this book, whether such damages are direct, indirect, punitive, incidental, special, or consequential.

Gregory Charlop, MD, is a practicing physician. However, this book does not establish a doctor-patient relationship. Dr. Charlop is not providing any medical advice in this book. Always consult your healthcare professional before deciding on any health, diet, or medical treatments.

This book does not provide financial advice. Dr. Charlop is not a financial advisor; no part of this book should be interpreted as financial advice. Always seek the advice of a qualified financial professional before any making financial decisions or investments.

Dr. Charlop is not a contractor, and the content within this book should not be used as a guide for home construction or modifications. Consult a trained professional or licensed contractor before any construction work.

The book contains several AI-generated images, notably in chapters 2, 5, 9, 10, and 14. These images are illustrative and should not be relied upon for accuracy or completeness. They are meant to provide a conceptual understanding rather than an actual representation of the topics covered.

Except for those in the introduction and conclusion, the narratives, characters, and scenarios presented in this book are entirely fictional. Any resemblance to actual persons, living or dead, events, or locales is entirely coincidental and unintended.

This book is provided 'as is' and reflects the author's views, knowledge, and understanding as of the publication date. It may not reflect current medical practices, building codes, financial markets, prices, rebate programs, or laws, which are subject to change.

This book may contain references to third-party entities, products, or services. Such references are for informational purposes only and are not intended to constitute, and should not be interpreted as, an endorsement, approval, or affiliation with any such third-party entities, products, or services by Gregory Charlop, MD, Dr. Greg LLC, or its affiliates. Likewise, these third-party entities have not endorsed or approved this book or its contents. Any trademarks or registered trademarks mentioned within this book are the property of their respective owners.

By reading this book, you acknowledge that you have read, understood, and agreed to this disclaimer.

About the Author

Physician and father of two daughters, Dr. Gregory Charlop (aka Dr. Greg), is passionate about sustainability and children's health. Since training at Stanford and UCLA, Dr. Greg has become a sought-after speaker, consultant, and nationally-recognized medical expert. Dr. Greg is regularly featured on major media outlets, including ABC, NBC, CBS, Forbes, and FOX.

Dr. Greg believes that human health and environmental sustainability are linked. Therefore, he helps families and businesses optimize their indoor spaces to promote health and productivity with an eco-friendly approach. His scientifically proven home rejuvenation formula protects the environment and supports radiant health.

Kids and pets are particularly vulnerable to unhealthy homes. Dr. Greg's expert tips can help clean indoor air, improve children's performance in school, and reduce the risk of childhood asthma and allergies. Plus, the kids will sleep better at night!

Struggling with fatigue or distraction while you're working from home? Dr. Greg's innovative use of light and design will enhance your productivity and creativity without medication. Get the natural edge you need to take your sleep and performance to the next level.

It's all here: *Dr. Greg's Green Home Makeover* is an easy-to-follow guidebook for a healthy, environmentally friendly, and productive home for your family. The book is based on Dr. Greg's extensive research and experience helping leaders remodel their homes for success.

Philanthropy is at the core of all of Dr. Greg's work. He allied with leading charities and social-impact investors to create From Soccer to C-Suite™, a multi-state leadership conference. His events support children's mental health and minority women entrepreneurs.

He founded the Women's Sports Forum series of conferences, podcasts, and events featuring powerful women athletes and business executives. He aims to inspire young girls to become leaders by sharing the stories of successful women.

Dr. Greg co-founded Electric Avenue Properties LLC, a syndicate that invests in sustainable properties near newly-announced electric vehicle and battery plants in Georgia and Ohio. His team supports community development to encourage the adoption of green transit and housing.

Concerned with global health and prosperity, Dr. Greg and his team are organizing an invite-only international consortium of business and thought leaders. The group promotes multinational networking and understanding.

Dr. Greg's last best-selling book, *Why Doctors Skip Breakfast: Wellness Tips to Reverse Aging, Treat Depression, and Get a Good Night's Sleep*, pulled back the curtain on anti-aging medicine and shared the simple steps we all can take to live longer, happier, and healthier lives.

If you'd like to request an in-person or video visit with Dr. Gregory Charlop and his team for your home or office, please reach out on LinkedIn or www.GregoryCharlopMD.com. He's available for speaking, consulting, or questions about environmentally sustainable homes.

Table of Contents

Introduction

July 10, 1976, the sun burned bright and hot in the serene Italian hamlet of Seveso. In this picture-perfect pastoral village, with roots dating back to the 3rd century BC, children sat down for a homecooked family lunch for the last time.

At precisely 12:37 p.m., an unearthly boom shattered the quiet town. It was a sound less heard than felt, a vibration that stirred the soul before the ears registered it. The ground bucked and roiled as if disturbed by some subterranean monster, and in the heart of the town, where the ICMESA chemical plant stood tall and menacing, hell opened its jaws.

With violent wrath, the manufacturing facility exploded, vomiting a cloud of dust that rose high into the blue sky. It bloomed like some grotesque flower, its petals a roiling mass of toxin-infused particles that refracted sunlight into a hundred unnatural hues. It was like watching a cobra uncoil and rise, the venomous fangs ready to strike.

A dark shadow rose in the sky over Seveso, filled not with rain but with the poison dioxin, an insidious harbinger of death. A silence swept over the town as the villagers looked up at their looming doom.

Then, the dust began to fall.

People ran, their voices thin and terrified against the backdrop of the still-settling explosion. Once a haven, their homes now stood beneath the descending cloud of poison. Panic spread faster than the dust, its tendrils reaching into every heart, every cottage.

It coated everything—skin, clothes, plants, roads, cars, and children's toys left out in the yard. It turned everything it touched into a dull, faded version of what it used to be, a still-life painting of a town under siege. It was a microscopic invader, a chemical alien that knew no barriers and respected no boundaries.

Then came the waiting, a dread-filled silence as the town held its breath, the ticking clock of doom echoing in their hearts. The dust had settled, but the effects, the true horror of what had happened, were beginning to crawl from the shadows.

First to fall were the animals, a pitiful omen of what was to come. Their vibrant eyes dulled, bodies twitched, then fell silent. Even the sturdy oaks and blossoming roses did not escape, their leafy green existence blackening under the silent assault of the invisible enemy.

The dust crept into homes, infiltrating the very sanctum of familial warmth and safety. From the hearty loaves in the baker's shop to the gingham tablecloths in country kitchens, the granules of death clung on, turning the familiar into vessels of fear.

And then it was the turn of the people. Like an insidious whisper, the toxin spread through their bodies, their skin erupting in a grotesque testament of its lethal potency. The eyes staring in horror at the unfolding catastrophe now streamed with tears, not of fear, but of physical torment. A miserable cough echoed through the streets, the once-robust voices reduced to raspy whispers.

Seveso, a name that once evoked images of pastoral tranquility and quintessential Italian charm, was now a symphony of sorrow. It was the embodiment of a town's descent into a horror story, its every corner, every stone, and every soul carrying the chilling narrative of a catastrophe that was neither natural nor distant.

The explosion at ICMESA was not just an industrial accident. It was a chilling prologue to a story that resonates today, a grim reminder of the dance on the knife's edge between progress and planet. It painted a terrifying portrait of an invisible war we wage against nature, a war that sometimes boomerangs back with a vengeance that forever scars the face of humanity.

Sometimes, the monster isn't hiding under your bed or in your closet. It can float in the air, invisible and deadly, its breath a poisonous whisper of extinction.

Following the Seveso disaster, Italian authorities and the community launched a massive cleanup operation. Over 700 people left their homes in the most affected areas. The cleanup crews had to remove tons of tainted soil. It took years to decontaminate buildings and public spaces.

In the immediate aftermath of the disaster, many people experienced severe skin conditions, the most common being chloracne, a type of acne directly associated with dioxin or Agent Orange exposure. Additionally, people suffered from eye inflammation, causing pain and making it hard to see. There was a surge in respiratory complications, with people struggling to breathe. Young and old, folks struggled with nausea, vomiting, and abdominal pain. The immediate health consequences were unnerving, but the future implications were downright terrifying.

The children of Seveso, growing up amidst the aftermath of the disaster, found themselves at an increased risk for a host of trouble. Learning difficulties increased, with many children struggling to keep pace with their peers academically. Additionally, they experienced motor skill impairment, which affected their ability to move, run, and jump. There was a rise in the incidence of specific diseases, such as thyroid disorders, abnormal weight gain or loss, fatigue, and mood disturbances. Cancer increased among the people exposed to the explosion, especially lung cancer and non-Hodgkin lymphoma. Girls exposed to dioxin often endured problems with their menstrual cycles and struggled to conceive later in life.

The disaster went beyond physical health. It had a profound impact on the mental and emotional well-being of the survivors. Many people, including children, had to deal with a lifetime of fear and stress because of the explosion and its aftermath.

We do not live in isolation from our environment. Our ecological missteps cause catastrophic and long-term consequences for animals and people. The more toxic stuff we buy to build, remodel, or furnish our homes and offices, the greater the manufacture of these dangerous chemicals. We ask for trouble whenever a factory belches out more unsustainable "goods." Our poor choices risk creating the next Seveso disaster. Make no mistake, the next poisonous cloud or toxic leak will come. It could be in your community or near the local water supply. And no amount of safety precautions or innovations will eliminate the risk of the next disaster.

Thankfully, there is something we, as consumers, can do. Cut back on products that depend on poisonous manufacturing processes. Minimize synthetic materials like vinyl flooring or toxic pesticides. There are healthier, natural alternatives. Read on, and learn how your greener home can protect the planet.

We owe it to our children and pets to make our homes safe. The hidden dangers in everyday items, like cleaning products, flooring, and cabinetry, often go unnoticed but can harm children's tender lungs. Mold and radon are silent threats, while a lack of natural light and fresh air can compromise your child's school performance.

As a physician with deep experience in restorative green home and office makeovers, I'm eager to guide you through your journey to a healthier and more productive life. I'll show you step by step what you must do.

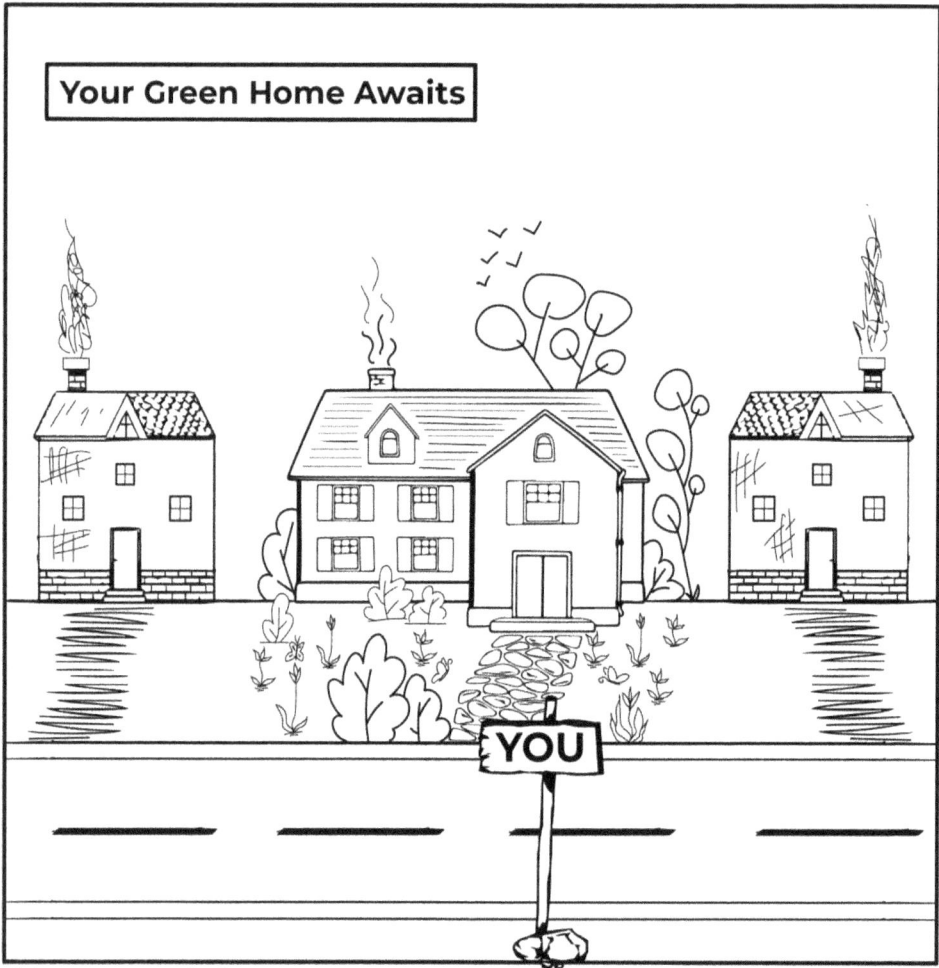

We spend so much time indoors. With careful planning, we can turn our homes and offices into sanctuaries that protect the planet, encourage productivity, and promote radiant health.

Sustainability starts at home. Now, let's get to it!

Dr. Greg's Green Home Makeover

Your Family's Guide to Healthy, Sustainable Living

CHAPTER 1

The World Is Burning, and So Are Your Kid's Lungs

Life was once idyllic and peaceful in the picturesque town of Lonesome Stables, surrounded by leafy forests and rolling hills. A young girl named Maria was proud of her home.

With a lanky frame and unlimited energy supply, Maria dreamed of becoming a gymnast. Maria practiced cartwheels and summersaults on her front lawn with her pup Lacy cheering her on.

But as the years passed, the world around them began to change. Industrialization and urbanization took a heavy toll on the town, poisoning the once-fresh air.

Clear blue skies slowly gave way to a hazy veil of smog as factories and automobiles pumped pollutants into the atmosphere. Giant energy-inefficient new houses invaded the quiet cul-de-sacs.

The town's air quality continued declining, and the residents started to suffer. Maria and her pup couldn't play outdoors because she'd cough and choke from the asthma and allergies she developed. She was constantly wheezing and struggling with school and gymnastics. Her grades took a nosedive.

Like other adults in the town, Maria's parents also began to experience health issues. Chronic respiratory problems such as asthma and bronchitis became commonplace. Productivity plummeted as people had to take more sick days to cope with their ailments. The fumes hit the elderly the hardest, as their weakened immune systems struggled to combat the effects of the bad air.

The town's residents, desperate for a solution, tried to fight the pollution. They planted trees and established green spaces. They installed air purifiers in their homes, hoping to reduce indoor air pollution. Yet, despite their best efforts, the air quality continued to decline, and the town's health issues persisted.

Lonesome Stables slowly fell into decay, its streets empty and buildings abandoned. The once-vibrant community crumbled as businesses closed and tourists stopped visiting, deterred by the town's sour air and scorched reputation. Maria's friends moved away, searching for healthier environments.

With a heavy heart, Maria's family decided they needed to leave their beloved town. Maria, her health continuing to suffer from the polluted air, was heartbroken to leave her home behind. Her dreams of becoming a gymnast now only a distant memory, she packed her belongings and said goodbye.

The story of Maria and her town is a stark reminder of the consequences of ignoring air pollution and its impact on our health and environment. Across the globe, air quality is getting worse, with more people exposed to hazardous levels of pollutants than ever before. The effects of this pollution on our health, as seen in this small town, are both widespread and severe.

As the world's climate changes and air pollution worsens, we must recognize the damage we're doing to our planet and take steps to mitigate it. We can protect our health, children's future, and the environment by transitioning to sustainable practices and green home remodels.

Children's health is deteriorating due to pollution

As pollution levels continue to rise, the most vulnerable members of our society – our children – are experiencing the worst effects of this environmental challenge. Exposure to air pollution can impact children's mental and physical health, shaping their future and overall quality of life.

Recent studies have found a strong link between air pollution and children's mental health, affecting their mood and cognitive performance. Research has shown that children exposed to higher levels of air pollution are more likely to develop cognitive difficulties, such as attention problems, memory deficits, and lower IQ levels. Moreover, air pollution has been associated with increased risks of developing anxiety, depression, and other mood disorders in children.

Living in polluted environments can exacerbate the symptoms of existing mental health disorders, making it more difficult for children to manage their emotions and cope with daily stressors. This emotional turmoil can ripple through their families as parents struggle to find support and resources for their kids.

Air pollution's impact on children's cognitive performance can have long-lasting consequences on their academic success and future opportunities. As they struggle in school due to attention and memory problems, their self-esteem may suffer, leading to difficulties connecting with their peers and forming meaningful relationships. Over time, these academic and social challenges can limit their potential and hinder their ability to thrive in adulthood.

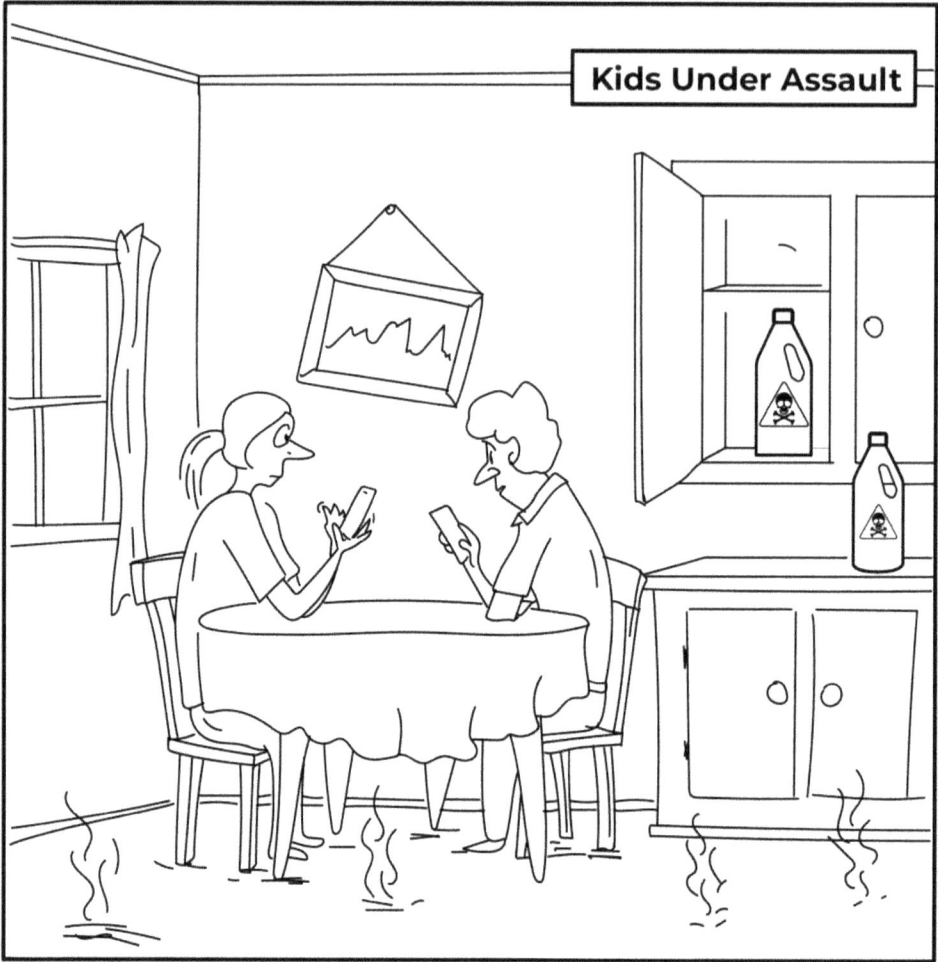

Visit www.GregoryCharlopMD.com

© Dr. Greg, LLC. 2023

Air pollution's impact on children's physical health is equally concerning. Children's developing lungs are more susceptible to damage from pollutants. Asthma is one of the most common chronic diseases in children and has been linked to exposure to air pollution. Other respiratory problems, such as bronchitis and pneumonia, are prevalent among children who live in polluted environments.

Smog can also harm children's cardiovascular and immune systems. Chronic exposure to pollutants can cause inflammation, leading to an increased risk of heart disease later in life. Air pollution can also disrupt the normal functioning of the immune system, making children more susceptible to infections and other illnesses. A weakened immune response can result in more frequent colds and flu.

Furthermore, research has shown that exposure to air pollution during pregnancy can negatively affect the developing fetus, leading to preterm birth, low birth weight, and other complications. Cleaning the air will help current and future generations of young people!

These children may face various health issues as they age, including chronic diseases and mental health disorders. The burden of these health issues affects individuals, their families, and society.

The story of Maria and Lonesome Stables is a poignant example of how pollution can devastate the lives of children and their families. As we continue to grapple with the challenges posed by air pollution, we must protect our children's health and well-being. We can create a healthier future for our children and the planet by adopting sustainable practices and investing in green home remodels.

The rise of cancer, asthma, harm to pregnant women, and Alzheimer's

Cancer:

Air pollution has been linked to an increased risk of various types of cancer, particularly in the lungs. According to the World Health Organization (WHO), outdoor air pollution is classified as a Group 1 carcinogen, meaning it has sufficient evidence to be considered a cause of cancer in humans. Pollutants such as particulate matter (PM), ozone, and nitrogen dioxide can damage DNA, leading to gene mutations that may result in the development of malignant cells.

Aside from lung cancer, air pollution has also been associated with an increased risk of other cancers, including in the bladder, breast, and gastrointestinal system. Reducing our exposure to air pollution can decrease the risk of these devastating diseases.

Asthma:

Asthma, a chronic respiratory condition affecting millions worldwide, has been strongly linked to air pollution. Pollutants such as particulate matter, ozone, and nitrogen dioxide can irritate the airways, leading to inflammation and constriction of the bronchial tubes. Inhaling these toxins can trigger wheezing, shortness of breath, and chest tightness.

Exposure to air pollution can exacerbate existing asthma symptoms and increase the likelihood of developing asthma in the first place. Children are particularly susceptible to the effects of air pollution on asthma, as their lungs are still developing, and their airways are more sensitive to irritation. By improving air quality through sustainable practices and green home remodels, we can reduce the prevalence of asthma and improve the quality of life for those living with the condition.

Harm to Pregnant Women:

Air pollution poses significant risks to pregnant women and their unborn children. Studies have shown that exposure to air pollution during pregnancy is associated with a higher risk of preterm birth, low birth weight, and intrauterine growth restriction. Fetal exposure to smog increases the risk of toddlers with chronic health conditions such as asthma, obesity, and neurodevelopmental disorders.

Pregnant women exposed to high levels of air pollution are at a greater risk of developing pregnancy-related health issues, such as gestational diabetes and preeclampsia. By clearing the air with energy-efficient homes, we can protect pregnant women's and their babies' health, ensuring a healthier start in life.

Alzheimer's and Air Pollution:

I bet you didn't see this one coming. Emerging research suggests that air pollution may play a role in neurodegenerative diseases, such as Alzheimer's and Parkinson's disease. Exposure to air pollution, particularly fine particulate matter (PM2.5), likely causes inflammation and oxidative stress in the brain, contributing to these debilitating diseases.

Some studies have found that living in areas with high levels of air pollution is associated with a higher risk of cognitive decline and dementia, including Alzheimer's disease. While more research is needed to understand the connection between air pollution and neurodegenerative diseases fully, these findings underscore the importance of addressing air pollution and adopting sustainable practices to protect our long-term cognitive health.

As the evidence linking air pollution to various health issues grows, it becomes increasingly vital for us to take action. Thankfully, you have this book to help keep you and your family safe!!

DR. GREG SAYS

Alzheimer's and air pollution

Air pollution and brain health are more connected than you realize. Scientists are now finding that dirty air might play a role in two major brain diseases: Alzheimer's and Parkinson's. Let's dive into what the latest research is telling us.

First, let's look at Alzheimer's, a disease where people slowly lose their memory and thinking skills. A study in the Journal of Alzheimer's Disease in 2020 found a link between dirty air and Alzheimer's. The problem comes from tiny pollution particles called PM2.5 that can sneak into our brains.

Once there, they create harmful changes that can lead to Alzheimer's. The idea here is that you breathe in these tiny pollutants, which get absorbed into your bloodstream and ultimately accumulate in and poison your brain. Yikes!

Studies from *Environment International* and other sources found a similar pattern. They looked at data from millions of older adults. For every slight increase in long-term exposure to PM2.5, the risk of Alzheimer's increased. This finding was true for many different groups of people, which tells us that this link between dirty air and Alzheimer's is likely real.

Now, let's turn to Parkinson's, a brain disease where people struggle with movement and balance. A study in the journal *Movement Disorders* in 2022 found a strong link between air pollution and Parkinson's. The main culprit is a pollutant found in diesel exhaust. These tiny particles damage certain brain cells that help control our bodies.

A study in *Environmental Research* focused on a different pollutant, nitrogen dioxide or NO_2. The researchers found that a slight increase in long-term NO_2 exposure could massively increase the risk of Parkinson's.

These tiny yet deadly particles often come from car and truck exhaust. Think twice about living near a busy roadway. And if you do, work with an environmental contractor to explore ways to seal out and eliminate these pollutants.

Animals are endangered due to deforestation, habitat loss, and climate change

Our actions profoundly impact the world around us, and one of the most significant consequences of thoughtless human development is the termination of countless animal species. Deforestation, habitat loss, and climate change contribute to declining animal populations worldwide. Here, we will discuss four specific examples that illustrate the plight of these animals and the importance of adopting sustainable practices to protect them.

1. Amazon Mammals:

The Amazon rainforest, home to an incredible array of plant and animal species, is threatened by deforestation and climate change.

A study by UC Davis found that a massive fraction of the Amazon's mammal species, including jaguars and giant otters, face extinction. As their habitats shrink and climate conditions become more extreme, these remarkable animals struggle to survive.

2. Coral Reefs and Marine Life:

Coral reefs, often called the "rainforests of the sea," support diverse marine life. However, these delicate ecosystems are susceptible to temperature and water quality changes, and climate change has led to widespread coral bleaching and reef degradation. As coral reefs fail, the many marine species that depend on them for shelter and food face starvation. Reef destruction will end the lives of countless fish, sea turtles, and invertebrate species, many of which are already facing the threat of extinction.

3. Polar Bears:

Polar bears are one of the most iconic symbols of the impact of climate change on wildlife. As global temperatures rise, sea ice in the Arctic is melting. This habitat loss has dire consequences for polar bears, which rely on sea ice to hunt seals, their primary food source. With fewer hunting opportunities, polar bears face starvation, leading to declining populations and a greater risk of extinction.

4. Monarch Butterflies:

Monarch butterflies, famous for their incredible annual migration, face numerous threats due to habitat loss and climate change. The destruction of their breeding grounds in North America, particularly the loss of milkweed plants, has led to a sharp decline in monarch populations. Additionally, extreme weather events and changing climate patterns disrupt their migration patterns, further threatening their survival.

These examples highlight the urgent need for sustainable practices and green home remodels to protect the health of our planet and its many inhabitants. By reducing our environmental impact, we can help preserve these vital ecosystems and the countless species that call them home.

You can make a difference

The challenges posed by air pollution, climate change, and habitat loss may seem overwhelming, but the good news is that we can make a difference. Sustainable housing and green upgrades offer a way to protect the environment, safeguard our health, and ensure a brighter future for all living beings.

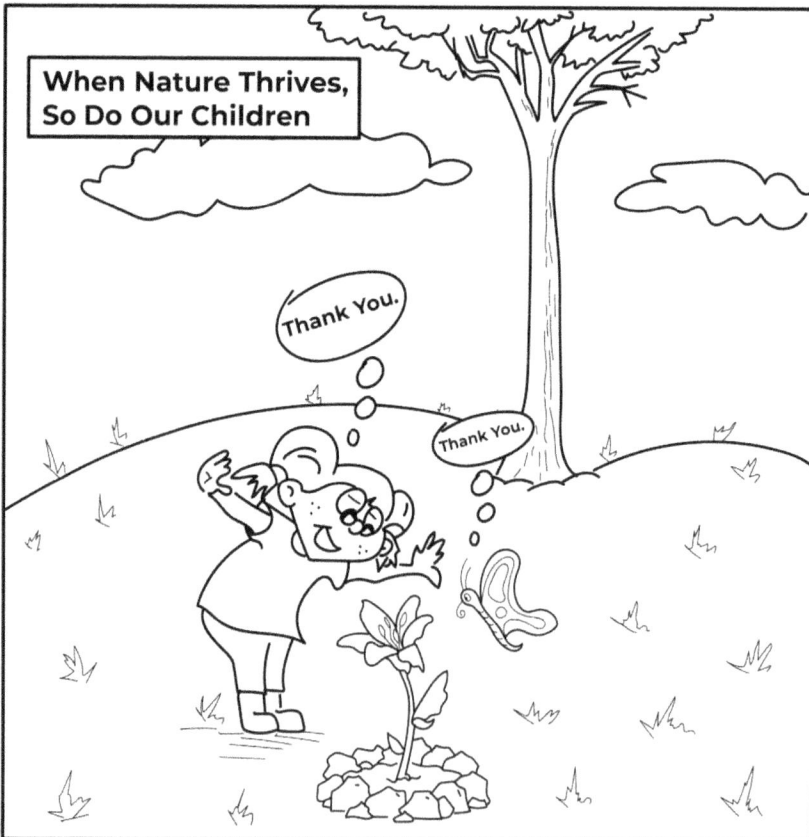

By making eco-friendly choices in our homes, we can reduce our energy consumption, decrease our reliance on fossil fuels, and minimize our production of harmful pollutants. Simple steps like improving insulation, installing energy-efficient appliances, and utilizing renewable energy sources like solar panels can significantly reduce the environmental impact of our homes.

In addition to the environmental benefits, green homes enjoy substantial cost savings. Energy-efficient homes require less energy to heat and cool, resulting in lower utility bills. Furthermore, many governments and organizations offer incentives and rebates to homeowners who invest in sustainable upgrades, making eco-friendly improvements an economically sound decision.

By choosing sustainable housing options, we improve our health and well-being and contribute to the health of the planet and its many inhabitants now and in the long term. Together, we can help reduce air pollution, combat climate change, and preserve vital ecosystems, ensuring a healthier, more sustainable future for future generations.

Interview: John Whyte, MD

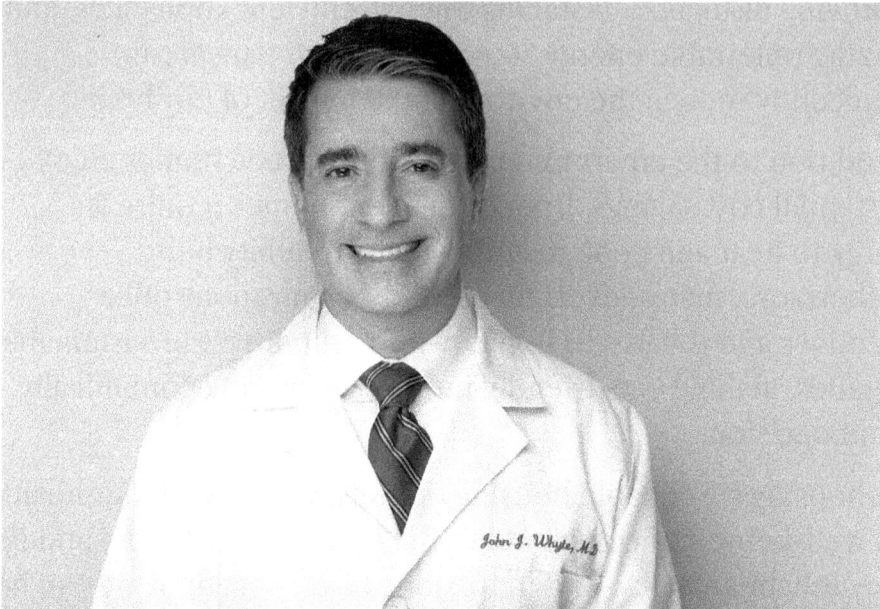

You'll enjoy my interview with Dr. John Whyte, my friend and the Chief Medical Officer of WebMD. We explored the intersection of building design, health, and productivity.

In today's fast-paced, digital world, we often overlook the importance of our natural environment, particularly when it comes to the places where we spend most of our time—our homes and workplaces. Science is starting to understand the crucial role that our environment plays in our well-being. Let's start with the impact of natural light on health and productivity. We tend to associate sunlight simply with vision, but it does much more than help us see. According to Dr. Whyte, "Natural light isn't just about visual comfort. It has far-reaching physiological effects. It regulates our body's natural rhythms—the circadian rhythms—influencing sleep patterns, mood, and even cognitive performance."

Top architects and designers integrate this knowledge into their work, crafting spaces that welcome natural light. "It's more than aesthetics," Dr. Whyte emphasizes, "Spaces bathed in natural light promote mental well-being, foster a positive mood and energy, and boost productivity."

For readers considering a new home, lack of access to morning light should be a deal-killer. Dr. Whyte explained, "When you don't have those natural light cues to respond to, it can disrupt your circadian rhythm. That can cause inflammation and an increased risk of cancer, diabetes, and heart disease."

The health-conscious design considerations extend beyond light. Clean water, for instance, plays a pivotal role. Buildings equipped with advanced water filtration systems can protect our health. As Dr. Whyte observes, "Water is our life source. Ensuring that this life source remains uncontaminated is one of the foundational stones of a health-promoting environment."

Our indoor environment can also harbor hidden threats. A notable one is mold. Dr. Whyte warns, "Mold can sneak into our spaces unnoticed. But its effects on our health are noticeable and can be severe, causing everything from allergic reactions to significant respiratory problems." Building designers and homeowners must ensure proper ventilation and moisture control to prevent mold growth.

The outdoor environment also impacts our health and productivity. "Engaging with nature, even if it's a small park or a landscaped area outside your office building, has a restorative effect," Dr. Whyte points out. "Several studies have indicated that spending time outdoors can improve concentration, inspire creativity, and lower stress levels."

Given the importance of outdoor spaces, it's great news that architects are finding innovative ways to integrate nature into building design. "We're seeing more green roofs, vertical gardens, and indoor-outdoor transition spaces. These are not just pleasing to the eye but act as stress-busters and productivity enhancers," Dr. Whyte remarks.

Resources like WebMD can help keep us updated on the latest wellness research. It makes complex information understandable. Dr. Whyte explained, "WebMD is dedicated to empowering people with knowledge that allows them to make better, informed decisions about their health."

Dr. Whyte said it best, "Good design is not just an art. It's a science that holds the potential to significantly improve public health."

John J. Whyte, MD, MPH

Physician/Executive/Strategist and Policy Expert

Dr. John Whyte is a physician and corporate executive with a unique combination of government and private sector work that provides him with an exceptional perspective on wellness, clinical trials, information technology, innovation, and health care services.

He is currently the Chief Medical Officer, WebMD. In this role, Dr. Whyte leads efforts to develop and expand strategic partnerships that create meaningful change around important and timely public health issues. He has been a leading voice in addressing the COVID pandemic, being named as one of the top 20 health influencers. Dr. Whyte is also a major contributor to iterating digital platforms from simply providing content, and instead playing a pivotal role in connecting to care. He frequently speaks on evaluating digital tools and technologies, assessing their roles in the evolving health ecosystem.

Prior to WebMD, Dr. Whyte served as the Director of Professional Affairs and Stakeholder Engagement at the Center for Drugs Evaluation and Research at the U.S. Food and Drug Administration. In this role, Dr. Whyte spearheaded numerous efforts to address diversity in drug development programs especially as it relates to necessary changes in clinical trial design.

This includes strategies around patient recruitment and acquisition, as well as the use of adaptive clinical trial design and master protocols. Dr. Whyte also helped provide regulatory insight into the potential uses of real-world evidence in regulatory decisions, especially around patient-focused drug development. Dr. Whyte led a research agenda around drug safety issues, including prescription and over-the-counter products.

Prior to this, Dr. Whyte worked for nearly a decade as the Chief Medical Expert and Vice President, Health and Medical Education at Discovery Channel, the leading non-fiction television network. Dr. Whyte developed, designed and delivered educational programming that appealed to both a medical and lay audience. He provided strategic direction, aligning medical and public health interests, viewer demands and corporate funding opportunities. This required the use of targeted multimedia marketing and building brand identity for new products.

Dr. Whyte also served in numerous leadership roles at the Centers for Medicare & Medicaid Services. While there, he formalized the process by which the Medicare program determines coverage decisions, including the criteria meant by "medically necessary and reasonable." He helped determine, evaluate and implement the national Medicare coverage policies on medical items, non-implantable medical devices, pharmaceuticals, and laboratory tests. He also oversaw an ongoing analysis of innovative treatment patterns and activities that improve health care outcomes. He is a recognized expert on various payment policies and models.

Dr. Whyte is a board-certified internist and continues to see patients. He completed an internal medicine residency at Duke University Medical Center as well as earned a Master of Public Health (MPH) in Health Policy and Management at Harvard University School of Public Health. Prior to arriving in Washington, Dr. Whyte was a health services research fellow at Stanford and attending physician in the Department of Medicine. He has written extensively in the medical and lay press, including three best-selling books.

Email: jwhyte@webmd.net

LinkedIn: https://www.linkedin.com/in/drjohnwhyte/

Interview: Adam Myers, MD

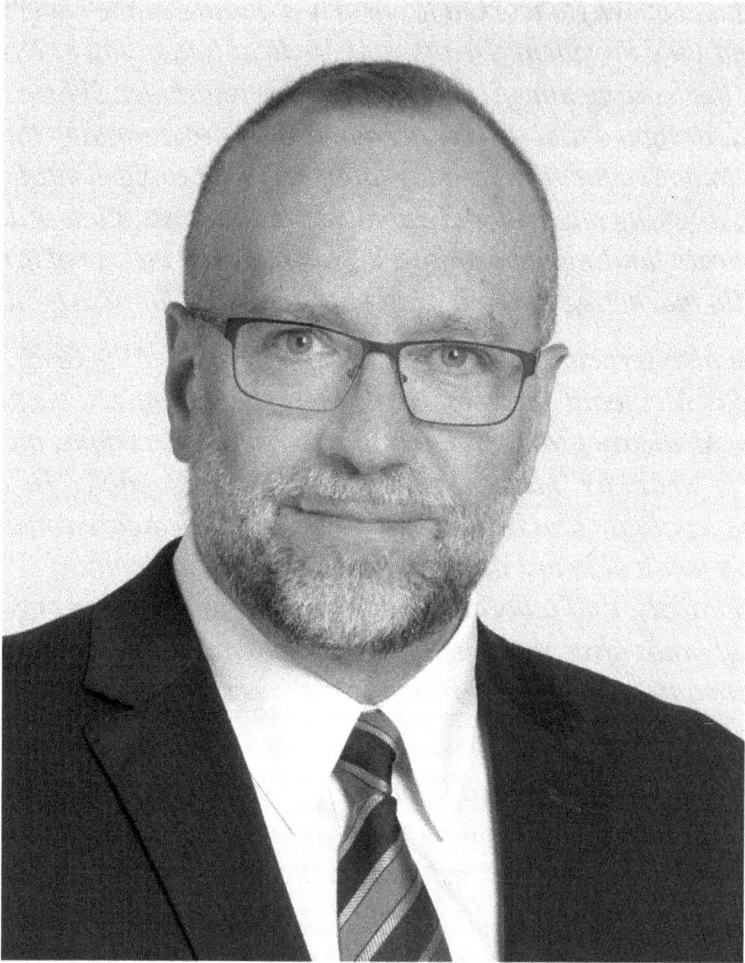

I had the pleasure of interviewing population health expert Dr. Adam Myers, the former Chief Clinical Executive at the Blue Cross Blue Shield Association, about the interface between housing, community, and human well-being.

Dr. Myers began by emphasizing the significance of natural light and green spaces for human health, even going so far as to prescribe outdoor walks to some of his patients. He explained, "People do well when there's good exposure to natural light and when there's access to green space. People just do well with that."

As our conversation shifted toward societal structures and their influence on health, Dr. Myers gave me a sobering perspective on lead poisoning and its correlation with housing conditions. He recounted his time at the Cleveland Clinic, grappling with high incidences of lead poisoning caused by decades-old paint, saying, "This is a health outcome that arises from a housing problem." In other words, proper housing powerfully influences our health.

It's in the interest of health insurers to encourage people to stay healthy. Dr. Myers said it well: The more health activities insurers are willing to cover, the more these activities will be implemented. "What gets paid for tends to occur, and what gets paid for more liberally tends to occur more often."

He praised Blue Cross Blue Shield for their regional management approach, community familiarity, and significant philanthropic funds dedicated to community health. Health insurers play a vital role in promoting health. He went on to mention the efforts of Blue Cross Blue Shield, which insures a staggering 115 million Americans, to encourage preventive care.

Our discussion led to the exciting Blue Zones Project—a collaboration between health insurers, local cities, and builders to enhance health outcomes. The initiative promotes community walkability, green spaces, access to healthy food, healthy habits, and municipal partnerships. Dr. Myers believes a society designed for activity encourages healthier, longer lives.

The conversation took a global turn as we discussed climate change and its repercussions on healthcare. Dr. Myers shared his anxieties about climate change-induced water shortages and deteriorating air quality. He shared a cautionary tale in Arizona, where climate change has led to severe water shortages in certain neighborhoods. "Water is a fundamental right," he said, "and seeing its availability threatened by climate change is not just an environmental issue; it's a public health crisis."

"You've got these homes in unincorporated areas that were developed and built, and people moved there under the impression that water would be available. And it's now clear those communities are quite literally drying up, and that's not good for anyone. The economic cost for those families is enormous as they then struggle to relocate when they discover they own a property that's not inhabitable."

Zooming back in on local issues, we discussed food deserts and the impact of diet on pregnancy outcomes. Dr. Myers said, "What people eat impacts their health... and certain diets, high in processed foods, and high-fat foods, are prone to produce hypertension, diabetes—which are some of the leading risk factors for adverse outcomes in pregnancies." The lack of access to healthy food is poisoning pregnant women and their unborn babies.

"People need access to produce and healthier foods that are culturally sensitive and taste good."

Dr. Myers highlighted the necessity for innovative solutions and partnerships between public and private entities in addressing these systemic issues. He shared an uplifting story from northeast Ohio about a successful collaboration introducing a grocery store to a previously classified food desert. He also shared the Fresh Fairfax initiative, which involves medical students visiting community members and creating healthier, culturally sensitive recipes.

Healthcare extends beyond the doctor's office, intertwining with various aspects of our lives—our living conditions, societal structures, and even global issues like climate change. This interconnectedness implies that our pursuit of better health should be as multifaceted and comprehensive as the issues we face.

Housing, nature, and community design are critical drivers of health. Thankfully, homeowners, government officials, medical professionals, and businesses can collaborate to make a meaningful difference in our lives.

———————

Dr. Adam Myers has the great fortune of having led in nearly every component of the health care delivery system. He is a frequent advisor, speaker, and advocate in key conversations at all levels. Most recently, he served as the Chief Clinical Transformation Officer for Blue Cross Blue Shield Association. In this role he drove clinical and operational transformation across the BCBS System serving 115 million members in the US alone. Additionally, Myers served as chief medical officer of the Blues' Federal Employee Program (FEP), which covers more than 5.8 million members across all 50 states and abroad. A longtime advocate for community health and health equity, Myers helps set the vision for the Blues' efforts to create a more equitable and affordable system of health focused on outcomes.

Prior to joining the Association in September 2021, Myers served as the Cleveland Clinic's chief of population health and director of the Cleveland Clinic Community Care program, where he provided leadership to a wide variety of clinical and residency programs, as well as the center for value-based research. In addition, he led the clinic's care model redesign strategy, their home care and virtual implementation strategy, the community and public health strategy, and the Diversity Inclusion and Racial Equity Council. Previously, he served in senior clinical and operational leadership roles at several large health systems, including Texas Health Resources, Southwestern Health Resources and Methodist Health System.

A New York City native, Myers is board-certified in family medicine and was in private practice in Oklahoma for more than 10 years. He served on the faculty of the University of Oklahoma obstetrics and gynecology department teaching obstetrics and has earned the status of Fellow with the American College of Healthcare Executives, The American Institute of Healthcare Quality and the American Association of Family Physicians. He holds additional board certification in healthcare quality management and patient safety and is a certified professional in healthcare risk management. He is past chair of the American Hospital

Association board-level Committee for Clinical Leadership and has held board positions with both the Health Care Transformation Task Force and The Joint Commission. He currently serves as a Health Evolution Fellow and is chair of their health equity initiative.

Myers received his undergraduate degree from Centenary College of Louisiana in Shreveport, where he graduated from Louisiana State University Medical Center. He completed his residency with In His Image Family Practice Residency at Hillcrest Medical Center in Tulsa, Okla., and completed fellowship in Advanced Obstetrics at the University of Oklahoma obstetrics and gynecology department. He also completed a master's in healthcare management from Harvard University.

On a personal level, he and his wife Melissa share 6 children and one absolutely adorable sheepadoodle named Pepper.

Email: adammyersmd@mail.harvard.edu

CHAPTER 2

Do Your Part:

Sustainable Building Materials

Deep within Brazil's Atlantic Forest, a family of golden lion tamarins thrived in their natural habitat. The patriarch, a strong and watchful father, and his mate worked together to care for their young offspring. These strikingly beautiful creatures, golden fur beaming like sunshine on a summer day, are marvels of the animal kingdom.

Golden lion tamarins lead a fascinating lifestyle. They are arboreal creatures, spending their lives in the dense forest canopy. As social animals, they live in close-knit family groups, cooperating in the search for food and shelter. They are frugivores, primarily consuming fruits, but they also diversify their diet with insects, small vertebrates, and nectar, which they find while foraging in the treetops. They play a vital role in the diversity of the forest ecosystem as seed dispersers.

The golden lion tamarins are sweet and loving parents. After a four-month gestation period, the mother typically gives birth to twins. Remarkably, the father takes on an active and nurturing role in raising the offspring, carrying the infants on his back and returning them to the mother only for nursing. This attentive care is essential for the survival of these tiny creatures, as they are vulnerable to predators and environmental dangers.

Unfortunately, the golden lion tamarins' idyllic existence is threatened by the rapid deforestation and habitat loss occurring in the Atlantic Forest. Once spanning over 1.2 million square kilometers, the Atlantic Forest has been slashed to a mere 7% of its original size due to logging, agriculture, and urban development. Tragically, the golden lion tamarin population has dwindled, with fewer than 3,200 individuals remaining in the wild today.

The plight of the golden lion tamarin is not unique. Today, more than 10,000 species are at risk of extinction in the Amazon alone, and deforestation is a devastating driver of this crisis. Forests worldwide are threatened, with dire consequences for the planet and its inhabitants. Deforestation contributes to nearly 20% of global greenhouse gas emissions and affects the planet's ability to regulate its climate.

We must acknowledge that the building materials used to construct our homes, schools, and offices can contribute to deforestation, habitat loss, and climate change. We, by extension, are helping to bring about the end of the golden lion tamarin.

But there is hope. By choosing sustainable building materials and practices, we can help endangered animals, safeguard the health of our families and pets, and save money on utilities and renovations.

How eco-friendly building materials protect the environment and your health

The use of eco-materials is not just a passing trend but a crucial step towards a sustainable future. By opting for environmentally friendly construction products, we can reduce our carbon footprint and protect vulnerable creatures, large and small.

When we choose eco-friendly materials, we help combat climate change by reducing the demand for resource-intensive products. Traditional building materials like concrete, steel, and aluminum require significant energy to produce and emit large quantities of greenhouse gases. Alternatives like reclaimed wood, recycled metal, or bio-based materials reduce our environmental impact and the strain on our planet's resources.

Eco-friendly building materials also help preserve biodiversity by reducing the need for logging, mining, and other extractive industries. For example, opting for bamboo flooring instead of hardwood can help protect forests and wildlife habitats. Bamboo is a rapidly renewable resource, growing up to 20 times faster than traditional hardwoods, and requires less land and water to cultivate. I can speak from personal experience. We installed bamboo floors in my home in the Bay Area and loved it. They stood strong against my busy young daughters riding their trikes all over the living room.

In addition to their environmental benefits, eco-friendly building materials can significantly improve the health and well-being of homeowners and their families. Traditional construction materials can emit volatile organic compounds (VOCs) and other harmful substances, which can cause respiratory problems and allergies. By choosing low-VOC, non-toxic alternatives, we can create healthier, safer living spaces for our kids and pets.

Some eco-friendly materials also offer excellent thermal insulation, reducing energy consumption and utility bills. For instance, materials like cellulose insulation, made from recycled newspapers (remember those?), or straw bale construction can provide superior insulation to conventional materials, keeping homes warmer in winter and cooler in summer.

Sourcing and certification - How do you know materials are eco-friendly?

Ok, ok, so I've convinced you to build and remodel with eco-materials. But how do you know what's legit and what's a scam? With the growing demand for green building materials, it's essential to identify genuinely eco-friendly products. Several certification programs and labeling systems can help ensure your chosen materials are sustainable and meet environmental standards.

Here are some examples of sustainable certifications to look for when sourcing building supplies:

1. Forest Stewardship Council (FSC): The FSC certification ensures that wood products come from responsibly managed forests, considering environmental, social, and economic factors. FSC-certified products help protect forests, promote responsible logging practices, and support the rights of indigenous peoples.
2. GREENGUARD: The GREENGUARD certification program, managed by UL Environment, evaluates building materials for their chemical emissions and indoor air quality impact. Products with the GREENGUARD label have been tested for low VOC emissions, helping to create healthier indoor environments.
3. Cradle to Cradle (C2C): The Cradle to Cradle certification assesses products based on their material health, material reutilization, renewable energy use, water stewardship, and social fairness. Products with the C2C certification are designed for a circular economy, where materials can be reused or recycled with minimal environmental impact.
4. ENERGY STAR: The Energy Star program, run by the U.S. Environmental Protection Agency and the U.S. Department of Energy, certifies energy-efficient products and materials, such as windows, doors, insulation, and roofing materials.

By choosing ENERGY STAR-certified products, you can reduce your home's energy consumption and save on utility bills.

With these labels in hand, you can build with confidence. The following sections will explore the best and worst options for flooring, cabinets, and countertops.

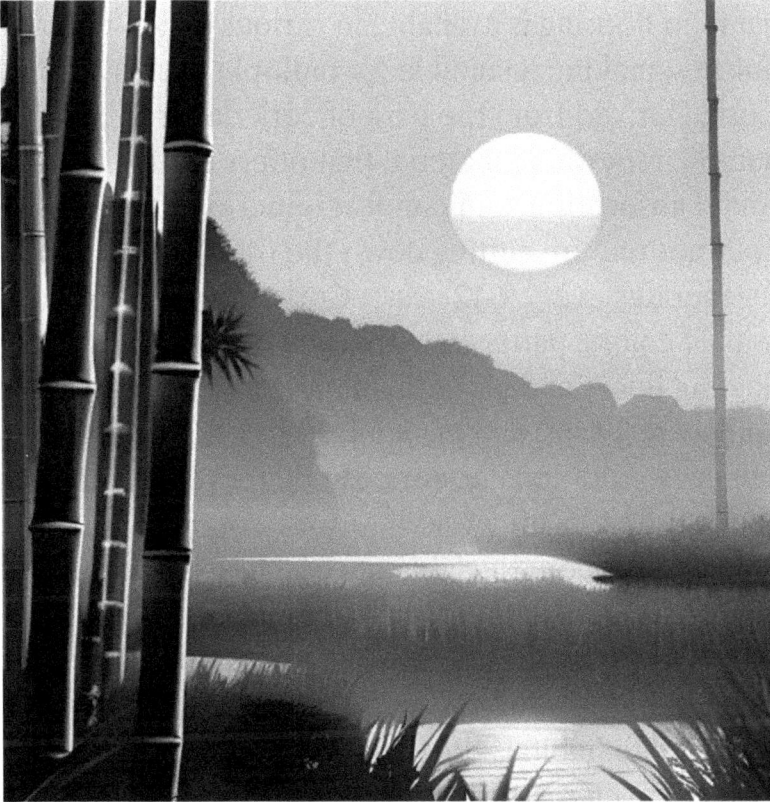

The best and worst flooring options

When selecting flooring for your green home remodel, it's essential to weigh the environmental impact and sustainability of each option. Here, we delve into the best and worst flooring choices, providing in-depth information to help you make informed decisions.

Best flooring options:

1. Bamboo: Bamboo is a rapidly renewable resource and a highly durable and versatile flooring material. It can grow up to 20 times faster than traditional hardwoods and requires less land and water to cultivate. It is easy to maintain and can be sanded and refinished like hardwood, ensuring a long-lasting, eco-friendly flooring solution. Moreover, bamboo flooring is available in various styles, colors, and finishes, making it suitable for multiple design aesthetics.

2. Cork: Derived from the bark of cork oak trees, cork is a natural, renewable material that offers excellent insulation, sound absorption, and comfort underfoot. Harvesting cork does not require cutting down the trees, as the bark regenerates every 9-12 years. Cork flooring is available in tons of colors, patterns, and installation methods, including floating floors and glue-down tiles. It is naturally mold and mildew resistant, making it a healthy choice for allergy sufferers. Additionally, cork can be recycled and repurposed at the end of its life cycle.

3. Reclaimed wood: Reclaimed wood flooring is the second life of salvaged lumber from old buildings, barns, and warehouses. By reusing existing wood, you help reduce the demand for new logging and contribute to preserving forests and wildlife habitats. Reclaimed wood flooring comes in various species, sizes, and finishes, offering a unique, rustic charm that can add character to any space. Before installation, it is essential to ensure that the reclaimed wood is treated and free of contaminants, like lead paint or pesticides.

4. Linoleum: Linoleum is a biodegradable, eco-friendly flooring option made primarily from linseed oil, wood flour, and cork dust. It is long-lasting, up to 40 years, and can be recycled once you're ready to move on to some new space-aged material. Linoleum is available in lots of colors and patterns, making it a versatile choice for various design

styles. It is also naturally antimicrobial, which helps maintain a healthy indoor environment.

5. Marmoleum: Marmoleum is a type of linoleum made with natural raw materials, including linseed oil, wood flour, and limestone. It is durable, biodegradable, and easy to maintain. Marmoleum comes in various colors, patterns, and installation options, such as sheet, tile, or click-together planks. Its antistatic properties make it resistant to dust and allergens, promoting a healthier indoor environment.

6. Recycled rubber: Recycled rubber flooring is made from post-consumer tires, reducing landfill waste and promoting a circular economy. It is slip-resistant, easy to clean, and offers excellent shock absorption and sound insulation. Recycled rubber flooring is available in rolls, tiles, or interlocking mats, making it suitable for various applications, including gyms, playrooms, and basements. One word of caution: rubber flooring may be inappropriate for folks with a latex allergy.

7. Recycled glass tile: Recycled glass tiles are made from post-consumer and post-industrial glass waste, offering a sustainable alternative to traditional ceramic or stone tiles. These tiles come in various colors, sizes, and finishes, providing a unique and eye-catching design element. They are durable, non-porous, and resistant to mold and mildew, making them ideal for kitchens, bathrooms, and other moisture-prone areas.

8. Natural fiber carpet: Natural fiber carpets, made from wool, sisal, jute, or seagrass, provide a sustainable alternative to synthetic carpets. Each natural fiber offers unique benefits, such as wool's natural insulation and flame resistance or sisal's durability and resistance to wear. These carpets are biodegradable, renewable, and often made with minimal chemical treatments, resulting in lower VOC emissions and improved indoor air quality.

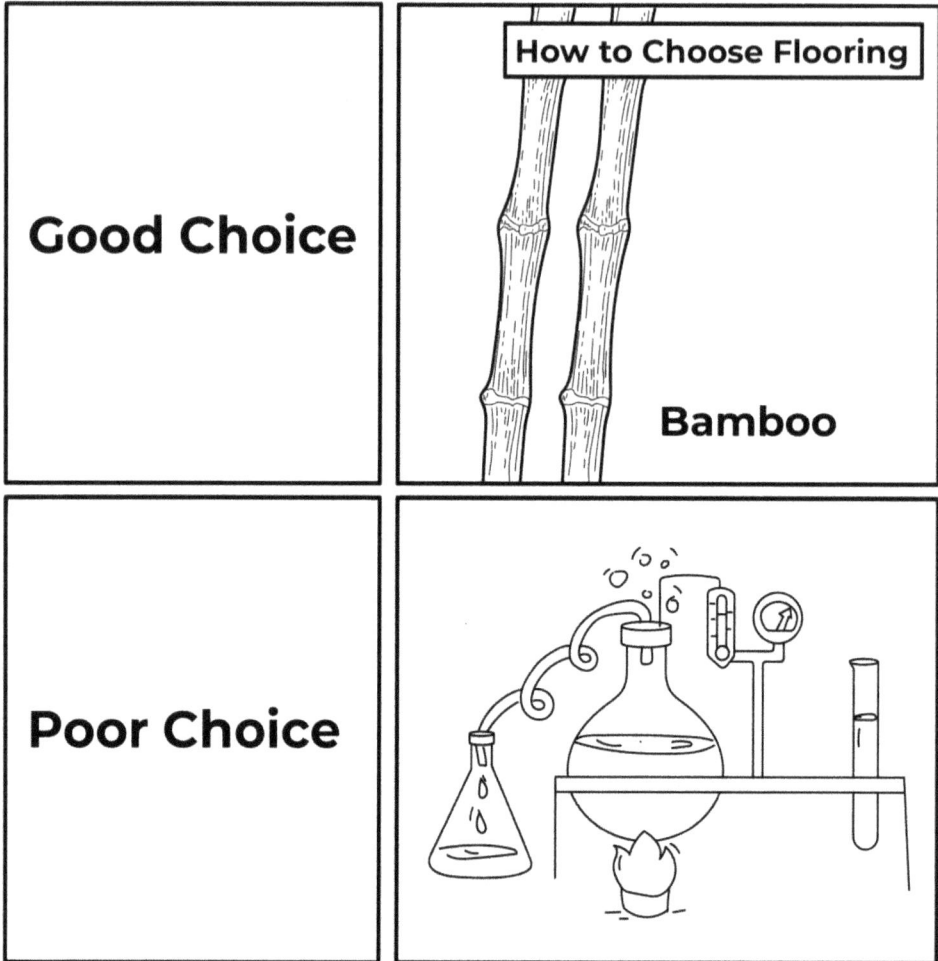

Good Choice

How to Choose Flooring

Bamboo

Poor Choice

Visit www.GregoryCharlopMD.com

© Dr. Greg, LLC. 2023

Use caution with the following:

1. Traditional hardwood: While hardwood flooring is a popular choice for its timeless beauty and durability, it can contribute to deforestation and habitat loss when sourced irresponsibly. When choosing hardwood flooring, opt for FSC-certified options or reclaimed wood as a more sustainable alternative.

2. Vinyl (PVC): Vinyl flooring, made primarily from polyvinyl chloride (PVC), is a non-renewable, petroleum-based material that can release harmful chemicals, including phthalates, during production and throughout its life cycle.

Vinyl flooring is challenging to recycle, often ending up in landfills where it can take hundreds of years to break down. If you're looking for a low-maintenance, water-resistant flooring option, consider eco-friendly alternatives like linoleum or Marmoleum.

3. Laminate: Laminate flooring consists of a fiberboard core topped with a high-resolution image of wood or stone, covered with a protective layer. While laminate flooring can mimic the appearance of natural materials at a lower cost, it often contains formaldehyde, a known carcinogen, in its adhesive layers. Additionally, laminate flooring is difficult to recycle and can contribute to landfill waste.

4. Synthetic carpet: Traditional synthetic carpets, made from nylon, polyester, or polypropylene, can emit VOCs and other harmful chemicals, negatively impacting indoor air quality. The production of synthetic carpets is also energy-intensive and reliant on non-renewable resources. When selecting a carpet, consider natural fiber options or look for carpets with eco-friendly certifications, such as the Green Label Plus from the Carpet and Rug Institute.

The best and worst cabinet and countertop materials

Like flooring, the materials you choose for your cabinets and countertops can significantly impact your home remodel's sustainability and environmental footprint. Here, we explore the best and worst options for cabinets and countertops.

Best cabinet and countertop materials:

1. FSC-certified wood cabinets: Cabinets made from FSC-certified wood are sourced from responsibly managed forests, ensuring minimal environmental impact. These cabinets are available in various styles, finishes, and wood species, offering a sustainable option for any kitchen design.

2. Bamboo cabinets: As a rapidly renewable resource, bamboo is an eco-friendly choice for cabinets. Bamboo cabinets are durable, moisture-resistant, and available in various finishes, providing a sustainable and stylish alternative to traditional hardwood cabinets. They're a great conversation starter, as few neighbors likely have these snazzy cabinets.

3. Reclaimed wood cabinets: Reclaimed wood cabinets utilize salvaged lumber from old buildings, barns, or warehouses, reducing the need for new logging and promoting resource conservation. These cabinets offer a unique, rustic aesthetic and can be customized to suit your design preferences.

4. Recycled metal countertops: Recycled metal countertops, made from post-consumer and post-industrial metal waste, offer a sustainable and stylish option for kitchens and bathrooms. These countertops are available in materials like stainless steel, copper, or aluminum and provide a modern, industrial aesthetic. They are durable, easy to clean, and can be recycled at the end of their life cycle.

5. Recycled glass countertops: Recycled glass countertops are made from post-consumer and post-industrial glass waste, creating a visually stunning and eco-friendly alternative to traditional stone or ceramic countertops. These countertops come in various colors, patterns, and finishes and are non-porous, making them resistant to stains and easy to clean.

6. Paper composite countertops: Paper composite countertops, made from recycled paper and non-petroleum-based resins, offer a durable and sustainable option for kitchens and bathrooms. Paper composite countertops are water and heat-resistant, making them a practical and eco-friendly choice. They are available in various colors and finishes, and you can sand or refinish them if they're damaged.

7. Quartz countertops: Quartz countertops, made from natural quartz, pigments, and resin, are an eco-friendly alternative to natural stone countertops like granite or marble. They are

non-porous, stain-resistant, and low maintenance, with lots of sparkly colors and patterns to match your taste. While not as sustainable as recycled materials, quartz countertops are a more environmentally friendly option than traditional natural stone countertops.

8. Bio-based solid surface countertops: Bio-based solid surface countertops, made from renewable materials like corn, soy, or sunflower seed oil, provide a sustainable alternative to traditional solid surface materials like Corian. These countertops are non-porous, resistant to stains, and available in various colors and patterns, making them an eco-friendly and stylish choice for kitchens and bathrooms.

Use caution with these cabinet and countertop materials:

1. Non-certified wood cabinets: Cabinets made from non-certified wood can contribute to deforestation, habitat loss, and other environmental issues. When selecting wood cabinets, opt for FSC-certified or reclaimed wood options to minimize environmental impact.

2. Particleboard cabinets: Particleboard cabinets, made from wood chips and sawdust bonded with formaldehyde-based adhesives, can emit harmful VOCs, impacting indoor air quality. Choose cabinets made from FSC-certified wood, bamboo, or eco-friendly materials.

3. Granite countertops: Although granite countertops are beautiful and durable, they can have a significant environmental impact due to quarrying, transportation, and energy-intensive manufacturing processes. Opt for more sustainable alternatives like recycled glass or quartz countertops.

4. Plastic laminate countertops: Plastic laminate countertops, made from layers of paper or fabric impregnated with melamine resin, are petroleum-based and can emit harmful chemicals. Additionally, they are difficult to recycle and contribute to landfill waste. Instead, consider eco-friendly

countertop materials like recycled glass, paper composite, or bio-based solid surfaces.

The Future of Sustainable Building Materials

As the demand for eco-friendly building materials grows, look out for some innovative new products. Promising developments in sustainable building materials include:

Biodegradable materials: Researchers are exploring the potential of biodegradable materials like mycelium (mushroom-based) insulation or bioplastics made from algae or bacteria. These materials can break down naturally, reducing waste and environmental impact.

Carbon-negative materials: Carbon-negative materials, such as carbon capture concrete or hempcrete, can absorb and store more carbon dioxide (CO_2) than they emit during production and use. By utilizing these materials, buildings can help mitigate climate change by reducing their overall carbon footprint.

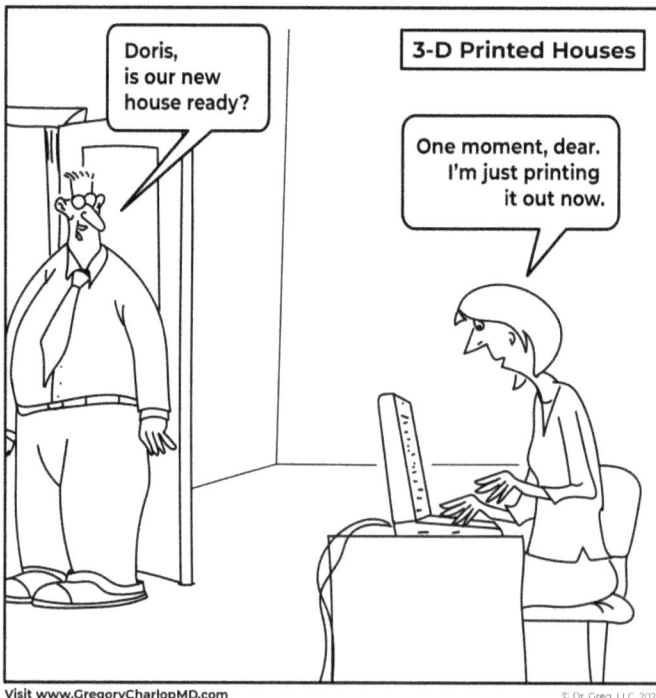

3D-printed construction materials: 3D printing technology has the potential to revolutionize the construction industry by reducing waste, lowering production costs, and enabling innovative designs. 3D-printed building materials can be made from recycled materials, such as plastic waste or construction debris, creating a more sustainable building process.

Modular and prefabricated construction: Modular and prefabricated construction methods can reduce material waste, energy consumption, and transportation emissions by manufacturing building components off-site in controlled environments. These methods can also facilitate using sustainable materials and energy-efficient designs, creating more eco-friendly buildings.

Next time you remodel your home, give these gems a try.

Interview: Stephanie Seferian

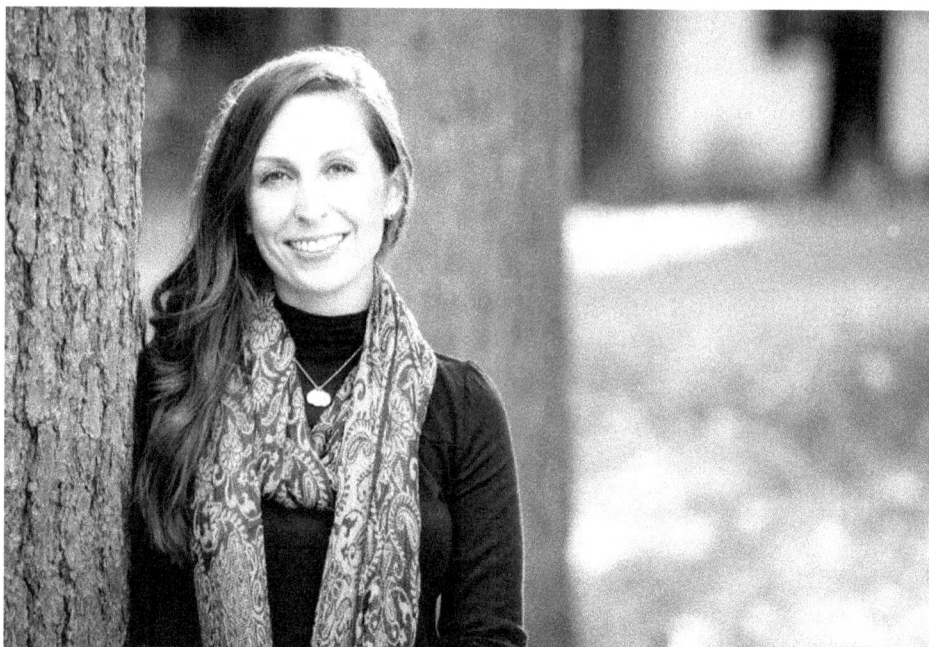

I had the pleasure of interviewing Stephanie Seferian, the thought-provoking host of the "Sustainable Minimalists" podcast and author of the book "Sustainable Minimalism: Embrace Zero Waste, Build Sustainability Habits That Last, and Become a Minimalist Without Sacrificing the Planet." Her refreshing perspective challenges our culture's obsession with more, more, more, advocating for a purposeful lean towards less. Stephanie's philosophy revolves around embracing a life of intentional simplicity that goes against the grain of our excessive consumer culture.

Early on, we dove into the controversial trend of ever-expanding home sizes that have become a status symbol in states like Texas and Nevada. Stephanie's stance on this trend was clear from the get-go. "A massive home isn't necessarily a sign of success," she argued, "but rather a symptom of our culture's encouragement of overconsumption." We are often tricked into thinking that the sprawling, 4,000-5,000 square foot house is a hallmark of 'making it,' when in reality, it might just be a monument to our inflated egos.

Digging deeper into this phenomenon, Stephanie highlighted a subtle but significant connection, "When you buy a larger house, you often tend to buy more unnecessary stuff to fill it," she observed. After all, you can't have an empty, unfurnished room! The consequence, she pointed out, is an endless cycle of accumulation that is neither sustainable nor satisfying. Her argument exposes the unseen side of the 'bigger is better' mentality that permeates our society.

Pivoting to the practical aspects of sustainable living, Stephanie offered some powerful insights. She challenged us to scrutinize the need for every potential purchase, citing a bread maker as a prime example of an unnecessary gadget that promises convenience but often collects dust. "If you don't bake bread weekly, you don't need a bread maker. Simple as that. We need to stop buying things because they're marketed as easy solutions," she commented, emphasizing the importance of differentiating between what we want and what we need.

Her ethos of intentional living was a recurring theme throughout our conversation. Stephanie pointed out that a minimal lifestyle doesn't equate to deprivation. Instead, it's about making conscious decisions that align with our values. "Minimalism isn't about living in an empty house," she remarked, "It's about surrounding yourself with the things that you love and truly need, discarding the rest."

We also explored the concept of self-sufficiency as an antidote to consumerism. Stephanie drew on the seemingly small act of hanging clothes out to dry as an example. Besides the clear environmental benefits of air-drying, she pointed out a lesser-known advantage: it helps preserve the longevity of our clothes. "Using a dryer isn't just energy inefficient; it also degrades your clothes," she noted. When expanded to other facets of our lives, this simple tip can significantly reduce our dependency on energy-consuming appliances and our overall environmental impact.

Throughout our discussion, Stephanie kept reverting to the idea that sustainable minimalism is an ongoing journey, not a destination. "The change won't happen overnight," she warned, "It's a gradual process. Every small decision to live more sustainably or to say no to unnecessary consumption adds up." She advocates for a thoughtful approach, where we regularly examine our habits, ask ourselves hard questions, and strive to align our actions with our values.

Stephanie's podcast, "Sustainable Minimalists," offers a deeper dive into these principles. Through thought-provoking discussions and practical advice, she encourages listeners to challenge societal norms and work towards a lifestyle that prioritizes sustainability over consumption.

Stephanie's insights into sustainable minimalism are not just food for thought but a call to action. Her work reminds us of our potential to disrupt the culture of excess, embrace intentional living, and foster a more sustainable future. Whether it's questioning the need for a bigger house, scrutinizing every purchase, or rethinking our laundry habits, Stephanie's message challenges us to reclaim control of our lives from the grasp of consumerism.

Stephanie Seferian is the host of The Sustainable Minimalists podcast; she's also the author of the non-fiction book Sustainable Minimalism. Stephanie lives just outside of Boston with her two daughters, yellow Labrador Retriever, 10,000-ish bees, and husband who loves to compost almost as much as she.

Instagram: https://www.instagram.com/sustainableminimalists/
Website: https://www.mamaminimalist.com

CHAPTER 3

Watch Your Breath:

Indoor Air Quality

Ella, a ten-year-old with an explorer's heart, lived smack dab in the middle of a leafy neighborhood that looked like it had jumped right off a postcard. A kid with more questions than stars in the sky, you'd usually catch her in the woods behind her family's old Victorian house, climbing trees and pocketing shiny things she found. And her room? Well, it was practically a zoo, thanks to her soft spot for nursing hurt animals back to health.

Mia and Tom, Ella's folks, thought the world of their kid and her kind-hearted nature. They didn't just put up with her animal-saving antics—they celebrated them. But there was a gnawing worry that kept them up at night. Ella's asthma and allergies didn't play nicely with their vintage house, and her wheezing and sneezing fits came more often, especially when the moon was up. It wasn't just costing her sleep—it was making it tough for her to stay focused in school.

Poring over the advice of doctor after doctor, Mia and Tom tried a laundry list of meds and treatments, but none of them hit the mark. They started to wonder if their beloved old house was part of the problem.

Mia, ever the researcher, stumbled upon an article that made her see things in a new light. It was all about the air inside our homes and how it can mess with our health. The thought had never crossed their minds, but now it was all they could think about. They didn't want their active little girl sidelined.

Indoor air quality isn't just about whether your house smells like fresh laundry or last night's takeout. It's about the stuff in the air that you can't see—things that can make you sick, especially if you already have lung issues. The EPA says we spend about 90% of our time inside, where there can be two to five times as many pollutants as outside.

The usual suspects? Dust, mold, pet hair, chemicals that hang around in the air, and radon. They can come from anywhere— cleaning products, building materials, even the fresh air that sneaks in through the cracks. And when you combine lousy ventilation, too much moisture, and high humidity, you have a recipe for a real indoor pollution problem.

The more Mia and Tom dug into it, the more they realized they had to do something. They needed to clean up their act and air for Ella's sake. And so they promised each other: they would do whatever it took to make their home a healthier place to breathe. And just like that, they were off on their next big adventure.

In the following sections, we'll delve deeper into the factors contributing to poor indoor air quality, how it can affect physical and mental health, and strategies to improve air quality within your home. Understanding these concepts and implementing a few household changes can create a healthier living space for you and your loved ones.

The top ten factors that contribute to poor indoor air quality

As we learned from Ella's story, indoor air quality is crucial in maintaining a healthy living environment. To better understand how to improve the air quality within your home, let's examine the top ten factors that contribute to poor indoor air quality:

1. Dust and allergens: Dust particles and allergens such as pollen, pet dander, and dust mites are common indoor air pollutants. They accumulate on surfaces and be released into the air when disturbed, leading to allergic reactions and respiratory issues for sensitive individuals.

2. Mold and mildew: Excess moisture, high humidity, and poor ventilation promote mold and mildew growth. Yuck! Exposure to mold spores can trigger allergic reactions and respiratory problems, especially for those with pre-existing conditions like asthma.

3. Volatile Organic Compounds (VOCs): These are gases that drift off certain building materials, furnishings, paint, and household cleaning products. Prolonged VOC exposure can cause eye, nose, and throat irritation, headaches, and even liver, kidney, and central nervous system damage.

4. Radon: Radon is a naturally occurring radioactive gas that can seep into homes through cracks in the foundation or other openings. Long-term exposure to high radon levels can increase the risk of lung cancer. Since it is odorless and colorless, the trick here is catching the radon with specialized tests.

5. Tobacco smoke: Secondhand smoke from tobacco products contains numerous harmful chemicals and can be particularly dangerous for children, pregnant women, and those with respiratory conditions. It can increase the risk of respiratory infections, asthma attacks, cancer, and sudden infant death syndrome (SIDS).

6. Carbon monoxide (CO): A colorless, odorless gas produced by burning fuel in cars, small engines, stoves, fireplaces, and other appliances. Exposure to high levels of CO can lead to headaches, dizziness, vomiting, and even death.

7. Pesticides: Indoor use of pesticides can introduce toxic chemicals into the air, leading to various health problems, including headaches, dizziness, and respiratory issues.

8. Biological contaminants: Bacteria, viruses, and other microorganisms can enter the home through various sources, such as people, pets, and outdoor air. Poor ventilation and high humidity levels can create an ideal environment for these contaminants to thrive, increasing the risk of infections and illnesses.

9. Asbestos: Asbestos is a naturally occurring mineral fiber used in many building materials and products due to its strength and resistance to heat. When asbestos-containing materials are damaged or disturbed, asbestos fibers can be released into the air, potentially leading to lung cancer, mesothelioma, and other serious health problems. The US banned this toxin in 1989, but it still exists in many older homes.

10. Lead: Although lead-based paint was banned in the United States in 1978, many older homes still contain lead in their paint, dust, and soil. Even at low levels, lead exposure can cause serious health problems, particularly for children, including learning disabilities, behavioral issues, and impaired growth.

DR. GREG SAYS

Secondhand smoke

This book talks a lot about indoor air quality, but one contaminant is worse than all the rest: secondhand smoke. This invisible toxin, the product of burning tobacco and exhaled smoke, poisons the air with over 7,000 chemicals. Of these, around 70 have been identified as carcinogens—agents capable of causing cancer.

Regular exposure precipitates the development of coronary heart disease, leading to a 25-30% higher risk than those unexposed. The smoke's toxic elements can induce arterial damage, contributing to plaque build-up and ultimately escalating the likelihood of heart attacks and other heart-related complications.

Secondhand smoke significantly threatens lung health too. Folks exposed to it suffer from a dramatic increase in lung cancer risk. This nasty, uninvited guest introduces tons of carcinogens into the body, causing DNA damage in lung cells. Smoke exposure is one of the prime causes of chronic obstructive pulmonary disease (COPD).

It's not just a matter of health. The productivity costs of exposure to secondhand smoke are substantial. Workers subjected to secondhand smoke tend to miss more workdays due to related illnesses compared to their smoke-free counterparts. The result? Higher absenteeism rates and the consequential negative impact on work performance and efficiency.

Finally, there's even a link between secondhand smoke exposure and the flu! The smoke compromises the immune system, rendering those exposed more susceptible to viral infections like influenza. Children living with smokers have more frequent and severe flu episodes. Not good.

But secondhand smoke isn't the only concern. There's even something called thirdhand smoke. This refers to the tobacco smoke residue that clings to clothing, furniture, and other surfaces. Not only can it be inadvertently inhaled, but it can also be ingested or absorbed through the skin, posing a particular danger to children or pets who may touch contaminated surfaces and then put their hands in their mouths.

So, what's your shield against this invisible enemy? Smoking outside doesn't cut it since smoke can waft back in through windows or doors. Air purifiers, while efficient at filtering particles, can't completely remove gaseous pollutants like those in tobacco smoke. Your best bet? Make your home a smoke-free fortress. Don't smoke. If you must, smoke far from the house, wear a smoking jacket, and deep clean surfaces to eliminate thirdhand smoke. Ventilate well.

Secondhand smoke is an insatiable killer; it seeps everywhere, indifferent to the borders of your apartment. Studies have shown that secondhand smoke can migrate between units in multi-unit buildings. That means you could be involuntarily inhaling your neighbor's smoke even if you're not lighting up.

So, to the managers of apartment complexes, a plea: it's time to enforce smoke-free policies in your buildings. The harmful effects of secondhand smoke don't respect property boundaries, so we must take measures to protect all residents. Restrict smoking to certain buildings or, better yet, ban it altogether. That way, you'll prioritize public health and safeguard our homes.

Eight ways poor indoor air quality harms physical and mental health

Poor indoor air quality can significantly affect physical and mental health. Here are eight ways poor indoor air quality can harm you and your family:

1. Respiratory issues: Exposure to dust, allergens, mold, and secondhand smoke can irritate the respiratory system, leading to coughing, wheezing, shortness of breath, and worsening asthma symptoms. The irritation caused by these pollutants can damage the lining of the airways, making them more susceptible to infections and inflammation. Long-term exposure to these pollutants can increase the risk of developing chronic respiratory diseases like chronic obstructive pulmonary disease (COPD) and bronchitis. In children, exposure to indoor air pollutants may trigger asthma attacks and increase the risk of catching the flu.

2. Allergies: Common indoor allergens, like pollen, pet dander, and dust mites, can trigger allergic reactions in sensitive individuals. Symptoms may include sneezing, itchy eyes, runny nose, and skin rashes. Prolonged exposure to allergens can also contribute to developing allergic asthma. Allergic reactions occur when the immune system overreacts to a substance, releasing histamine and other chemicals that cause inflammation and allergy symptoms. Exposure to indoor allergens can sensitize the immune system, increasing the likelihood of developing allergies to other things.

3. Cardiovascular problems: Airborne particles, such as those found in tobacco smoke and certain indoor air pollutants, can be inhaled deep into the lungs, potentially causing inflammation and damage to the cardiovascular system. When inhaled, fine particles can enter the bloodstream, leading to systemic inflammation and oxidative stress, damaging blood vessels and promoting blood clots. Additionally, exposure to high levels of indoor air pollution can cause an imbalance in the autonomic nervous system, resulting in increased heart rate and blood pressure. This inflammatory state increases the risk of heart attack and stroke.

4. Cognitive impairment: Exposure to high levels of indoor air pollutants like carbon monoxide, lead, and certain VOCs can impair cognitive function, leading to difficulties with concentration, memory, and decision-making. Carbon monoxide can interfere with the brain's ability to utilize oxygen, while lead exposure can damage the developing nervous system in children, leading to learning disabilities and behavioral problems. VOCs, such as formaldehyde and benzene, can affect the central nervous system, potentially causing cognitive and neurological impairments. Additionally, prolonged exposure to high levels of indoor air pollution has been linked to an increased risk of developing

neurodegenerative diseases like Alzheimer's and Parkinson's.

5. Headaches and fatigue: Poor indoor air quality can cause headaches, fatigue, and dizziness, particularly when pollutants like VOCs, carbon monoxide, and mold are present. Nasties in the air may dilate blood vessels in the brain and trigger headaches. Fatigue may result from the body's efforts to detoxify and eliminate harmful substances inhaled from the air, placing additional strain on the immune system and leaving the individual feeling drained and exhausted. Dizziness can occur when the brain is deprived of oxygen, as in the case of carbon monoxide exposure, or due to the effects of certain VOCs on the central nervous system.

6. Irritation of the eyes, nose, and throat: Many indoor air pollutants can irritate the eyes, nose, and throat. Prolonged exposure to these irritants can lead to chronic inflammation, potentially resulting in sinusitis, rhinitis, and pharyngitis. Some VOCs and particulate matter can even cause damage to the delicate mucous membranes lining the eyes, nose, and throat, making them more susceptible to infections and other health issues.

7. Increased risk of infections: Poor indoor air quality can compromise the immune system, making individuals more susceptible to infections, such as colds, flu, and other respiratory illnesses. Exposure to biological contaminants, such as bacteria, viruses, and mold, can stimulate the immune system, potentially causing it to become overactive or less effective at fighting infections. Also, harmful chemicals and pollutants can weaken the immune system's ability to respond effectively, making the individual more vulnerable to illness.

8. Mental health issues: Studies have shown that poor indoor air quality can contribute to mental health challenges, such as anxiety, depression, and stress. There are several possible

mechanisms through which poor indoor air quality can impact mental health. First, the physical effects of air pollution on the body can cause inflammation and oxidative stress, which have been linked to the development of mental health disorders. Second, the psychological impact of living in an unhealthy environment can increase stress levels, potentially exacerbating existing mental health issues or predisposing individuals to develop new ones. Furthermore, research has shown that exposure to indoor air pollutants, such as VOCs, can directly affect mood and cognitive function. These pollutants can disrupt the balance of neurotransmitters in the brain, potentially leading to irritability, mood swings, and difficulty concentrating. In children, exposure to indoor air pollutants has been linked to behavioral problems and impaired cognitive development, which can have long-term consequences on their mental health and academic performance.

Another aspect of the relationship between indoor air quality and mental health is the impact of poor ventilation on cognitive function and mood. In some cases, poor ventilation can even lead to a condition known as "sick building syndrome," in which occupants experience a range of symptoms, including headaches, fatigue, and respiratory issues, that are alleviated upon leaving the building.

Poor indoor air quality can have wide-ranging effects on physical and mental health. The following section will explore practical strategies for improving indoor air quality and safeguarding your family's health.

DR. GREG SAYS

Air purifiers

Air purifiers are not just devices with sleek aesthetics; they're your home's personal bouncers, kicking out those unwanted, invisible irritants that trash your indoor air quality. But how do they do it, what should you look for when choosing one, and can they help with asthma, allergies, flu, and mold?

Air purifiers work by capturing and neutralizing particles you'd rather not breathe. The gold-standard HEPA (High-Efficiency Particulate Air) filters are particularly adept at this task, trapping up to 99.97% of particles as small as 0.3 microns. Since most of us have no clue how small a micron is, here's a fun fact: a single strand of human hair is about 70 microns wide. So, we're talking about tiny air particles!

Choosing an air purifier isn't as simple as picking the one that matches your curtains. You should consider room size, the device's clean air delivery rate (CADR), and the pollutants you want to remove. Consider a purifier with activated carbon filters if you're after gaseous contaminants like volatile organic compounds (VOCs).

Some air purifiers come with an ultraviolet light feature. These typically work by beaming UV-C light onto a portion of air flowing through the filter. Since UV-C is pretty strong stuff, it will theoretically kill some bacteria and viruses floating in the air. Unfortunately, there is very little evidence of benefit from this technology for home use, and it can produce ozone, which harms indoor air quality.

Regarding asthma and allergies, air purifiers can be valuable allies. A study published in the Journal of Allergy and Clinical Immunology found that air purifiers reduced levels of fine particulates in homes by around 50%, significantly improving allergic symptoms. But remember, an air purifier is not a silver bullet. It should be part of a broader strategy, including controlling allergen sources (like your beloved Fido or a dusty carpet) and ensuring good ventilation.

Influenza, on the other hand, is a tricky foe. The flu virus is tiny—small enough to slip through many purifier filters. I looked into this, and unfortunately, there's limited evidence that air purifiers can reduce influenza transmission. They don't hurt, but I wouldn't count on them to keep grandma safe if your daughter has the flu.

Now, let's tackle the subject of mold. These fungi can be a nightmare for your respiratory system; getting rid of them often requires more than just an air purifier. While these devices can capture mold spores, they can't tackle the root of the problem—moisture. That's where dehumidifiers come into play. You'll want to consult a mold abatement expert to eliminate that crud at the source. It's not a bad idea to use a dehumidifier and high-quality air purifier until your mold problems are solved.

Here's a surprising twist: air purifiers can unexpectedly benefit cardiovascular health. One study found that using an air purifier reduced PM2.5 (tiny airborne particle) exposure, significantly improving blood pressure. Now, that's a breath of fresh air!

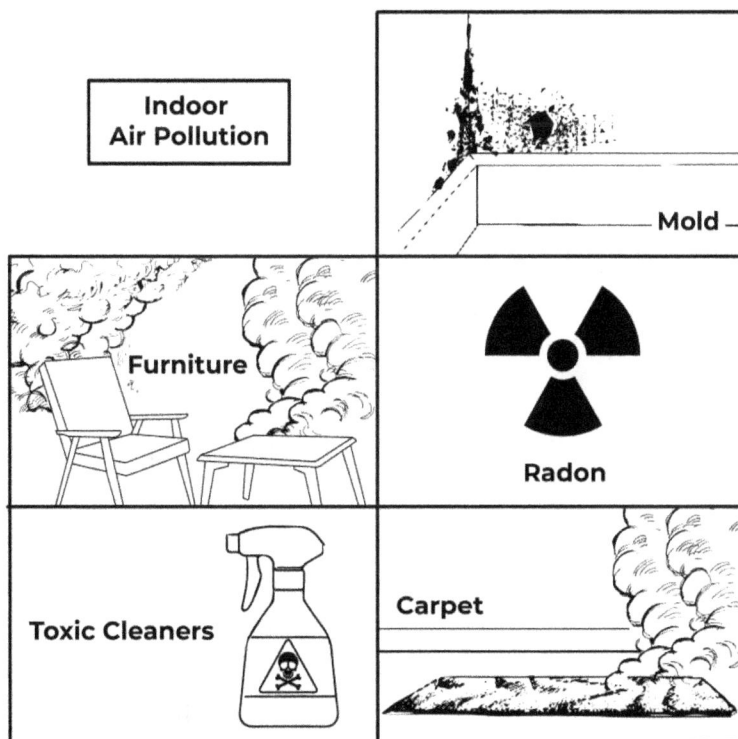

Indoor Air Pollution

Mold

Furniture

Radon

Toxic Cleaners

Carpet

© Dr. Greg, LLC. 2023

Twelve Strategies to improve air quality

1. Regularly clean and maintain your HVAC system: Ensuring your heating, ventilation, and air conditioning (HVAC) system is clean and functioning efficiently is crucial for maintaining good indoor air quality. Change filters regularly, clean ducts and vents, and have your system serviced by a professional as needed.

2. Use air purifiers: Air purifiers can help remove airborne particles, allergens, and pollutants from the air. Choose a purifier with a high-efficiency particulate air (HEPA) filter to effectively capture particles as small as 0.3 microns in diameter.

3. Control humidity levels: High humidity can promote the growth of mold and dust mites, leading to poor indoor air quality. Maintain indoor humidity levels between 30% and 50% using a dehumidifier or air conditioner. Dehumidifiers are essential in basements and crawlspaces.

4. Improve ventilation: Increasing the fresh air circulation in your home can help dilute indoor air pollutants and reduce concentrations of harmful substances. Open windows and doors when weather permits, and consider installing a whole-house ventilation system or an energy recovery ventilator (ERV) for a more energy-efficient solution.

5. Use exhaust fans: Properly functioning exhaust fans in kitchens and bathrooms can help remove moisture, cooking fumes, and other pollutants from the air. Be sure to use these fans while cooking and bathing to prevent the buildup of contaminants.

6. Choose low-VOC products: Volatile organic compounds (VOCs) pour out of many household products, such as paints, cleaning supplies, and building materials. Opt for low-VOC or VOC-free products whenever possible to reduce exposure to these harmful chemicals.

7. Properly store and dispose of chemicals: Properly storing and disposing of chemicals, such as paints, solvents, and pesticides, can help prevent the release of harmful fumes into your indoor air. Keep these substances in a well-ventilated area, away from living spaces, and follow disposal instructions provided by the manufacturer or local waste management authorities.

8. Keep your home clean: Regular cleaning can help reduce the accumulation of dust, allergens, and other pollutants in your home. Vacuum frequently using a vacuum cleaner with a HEPA filter, dust surfaces with a damp cloth, and wash bedding and curtains regularly to minimize allergens.

9. Maintain a smoke-free home: Secondhand smoke is a significant indoor air pollutant and can cause respiratory issues, heart disease, and other health problems. Quit smoking, and don't let anyone else light up in your house! This is an obvious one, but likely the most important.

10. Test for radon: Radon is a naturally occurring radioactive gas that can cause lung cancer. Test your home for radon using a radon test kit. If levels are elevated, contact a trained professional to help you eliminate this deadly gas.

11. Address mold and moisture issues: Promptly address any signs of mold or moisture damage in your home to prevent the growth of harmful mold and the release of mold spores into the air. Fix leaks, properly ventilate bathrooms and kitchens, and use moisture-absorbing products in damp areas like basements.

12. Use houseplants to improve air quality: Some houseplants, such as spider plants, snake plants, and peace lilies, can help filter indoor air by absorbing pollutants and releasing oxygen. It's important to note that while houseplants are the most beautiful solution to poor air quality, they should not be relied upon as your only option. Be sure to combine their use with the other strategies listed above for the most effective results.

DR. GREG SAYS

Radon and carbon monoxide

In the quiet corners of your home, undetected villains—radon and carbon monoxide—conspire against you. These unseen, odorless adversaries silently dance through your indoor air, a waltz of potential devastation. To ensure the safety of our indoor air, we must first understand these elusive gases. Let's bring these silent foes into the light.

Radon, a naturally occurring radioactive gas, emerges from the decay of uranium in soil and rocks. Surprising fact: it's the second leading cause of lung cancer, right behind smoking. It creeps into homes undetected through cracks and openings without taste, smell, or color. The only defense? Testing. It's simple, inexpensive, and life-saving. Purchase a radon test kit from a hardware store, follow the instructions, and send it to a lab for analysis.

Mitigation is the name of the game with radon. Depending on radon levels, professionals may be required to route this toxic gas from beneath the house into the open air.

Signs of carbon monoxide poisoning mimic the flu sans fever: headache, fatigue, shortness of breath, nausea, and dizziness. But here's the chilling part, extended exposure can lead to brain damage or death. Protection comes in the form of carbon monoxide detectors, required by law in many areas. Install them near the kitchen and bedrooms, and check the batteries regularly.

Ensure proper home and garage ventilation and regular appliance maintenance to reduce the risk of carbon monoxide poisoning. Don't run your car in the garage. If your carbon monoxide alarms suddenly go off, scoop up the kids and pets, flee the house, and call 911 (in the US). This dangerous gas can quickly overcome you.

Take a good look at your home. Those cracks in the foundation might be more than just an eyesore, and that old furnace in the basement might be harboring a deadly secret. A few simple steps can make all the difference. Remember, these enemies are invisible. Your weapons are vigilance, knowledge, and proactive measures. Arm yourselves, and breathe easier.

Now, meet carbon monoxide, another silent intruder. This byproduct of burning fuels (think: gas appliances or wood-burning stoves & fireplaces) is hazardous at high levels. It's known as the "silent killer" because it's also colorless, odorless, and tasteless. Carbon monoxide doesn't play; in high concentrations, it can kill in as little as 5 minutes.

Signs of carbon monoxide poisoning mimic the flu sans fever: headache, fatigue, shortness of breath, nausea, and dizziness. But here's the chilling part, extended exposure can lead to brain damage or death. Protection comes in the form of carbon monoxide detectors, required by law in many areas. Install them near the kitchen and bedrooms, and check the batteries regularly.

Ensure proper home and garage ventilation and regular appliance maintenance to reduce the risk of carbon monoxide poisoning. Don't run your car in the garage. If your carbon monoxide alarms suddenly go off, scoop up the kids and pets, flee the house, and call 911 (in the US). This dangerous gas can quickly overcome you.

Take a good look at your home. Those cracks in the foundation might be more than just an eyesore, and that old furnace in the basement might be harboring a deadly secret. A few simple steps can make all the difference. Remember, these enemies are invisible. Your weapons are vigilance, knowledge, and proactive measures. Arm yourselves, and breathe easier.

Ten surprising household items that harm indoor air quality

Many everyday household items can negatively impact indoor air quality, potentially posing risks to your health. Here are ten surprising sources of indoor air pollution:

1. Scented candles and air fresheners: While they may smell pleasant, aromatic candles and air fresheners can release VOCs and particulate matter. Opt for unscented candles made from natural waxes, such as beeswax or soy, and consider using essential oil diffusers or natural alternatives for freshening the air in your home.
2. Dry-cleaned clothing: The chemicals used in the dry-cleaning process, particularly perchloroethylene, can off-gas

from your clothes and pollute the indoor air. Choose a dry cleaner that uses environmentally friendly methods, or air out your dry-cleaned garments outdoors before bringing them inside.

3. Plywood and particleboard furniture: Many types of pressed wood furniture, such as plywood and particleboard, can release formaldehyde, a toxic VOC. Look for furniture made from solid wood, or opt for products certified as low-emission by organizations such as Greenguard or the California Air Resources Board.

4. Carpeting: New carpets can emit VOCs, such as formaldehyde and benzene, into the air. Choose carpets with low VOC emissions or hard-surface floorings, such as Marmoleum or tile, to reduce exposure to these chemicals.

5. Cleaning products: Many conventional cleaning products contain VOCs and other harmful chemicals that can pollute indoor air. Choose non-toxic, eco-friendly cleaning products, or make your own using natural ingredients like vinegar, baking soda, and lemon juice. Some brands are better than others, so pick the healthiest option.

6. Non-stick cookware: Non-stick cookware, particularly those made with Teflon, can release toxic fumes when heated at high temperatures. Use cookware made from stainless steel, cast iron, or ceramic materials to avoid this risk. Then, wash your stainless steel pots in the dishwasher. It cleans better than you might think!

7. Gas stoves: Cooking can release nitrogen dioxide, carbon monoxide, and particulate matter into the air. Ensure proper ventilation when using gas stoves, and consider installing an exhaust fan or range hood to help remove these pollutants.

8. Photocopiers and printers: Office equipment like photocopiers and printers can emit ozone and VOCs. Opt for low-emission devices, and keep them in well-ventilated areas to minimize exposure.

9. Hobby supplies: Some hobby materials, such as paints, solvents, and glues, can release harmful fumes into the air. Choose low-VOC or water-based products whenever possible, and work in well-ventilated areas when using these materials.
10. Pet dander and hair: Pet dander, hair, and saliva can contribute to poor indoor air quality by triggering allergies and asthma symptoms. Keep your pets well-groomed, vacuum regularly with a HEPA-filtered vacuum cleaner, and wash pet bedding frequently to reduce allergens in your home.

How to assess the quality of your indoor air

Let's root out some of the bad players in your home so you can start breathing a little easier. To begin, regularly inspect your home for signs of moisture damage, mold growth, and excessive dust. Watch for water stains, musty odors, and visible mold, indicating your house has a problem.

A crucial aspect of assessing indoor air quality is monitoring carbon monoxide levels. Carbon monoxide is colorless, odorless, and tasteless, making it difficult to detect without a proper alarm system. Installing carbon monoxide detectors throughout your home can help alert you to the presence of this dangerous gas. These are inexpensive and well worth the investment.

Go ahead and test for radon. As mentioned earlier, radon is a naturally occurring radioactive gas that causes lung cancer. Use a radon test kit to determine if your home has elevated radon levels. If the results indicate high radon levels, do not pass go, and give your contractor a call.

Consider hiring a professional indoor air quality specialist for more comprehensive assessments. These experts can test various pollutants, such as VOCs, mold spores, and allergens, and provide detailed information on your home's air quality. Based on the test results, they can also offer guidance on how to improve indoor air quality.

Additionally, check out indoor air quality monitors--these devices can measure levels of pollutants like VOCs, particulate matter, and humidity. They can help keep track of your home's air quality in real-time. With these handy gizmos, you can track how effectively your remodels clear the air.

Lastly, don't underestimate the power of your senses. If you notice persistent odors or experience frequent allergy symptoms, headaches, or respiratory issues while at home, it could be a sign that your indoor air quality needs improvement. Trust your instincts and take action to address these issues, whether it's through improving ventilation, using air purifiers, or addressing sources of pollution.

Stay vigilant. Just like Mia and Tom, you can monitor and clean up your indoor air so your kids can breathe a little easier.

CHAPTER 4

Tiny Toxic Bubbles:
Common Household Dangers

In Maria's once minimalist, meticulously-decorated apartment, her daughter Sophie brought an explosion of color and chaos. With bright green eyes always looking for her next adventure, the one-year-old redhead turned her mom's orderly world upside down. Instead of quiet architectural drawings, their quiet space now buzzed with Sophie's beeping toys, books ready for teething, and Daisy, her slightly ragged yet beloved bunny.

The family had a ritual. After finishing work designing a local office park or restaurant each evening, Maria would dutifully scrub down her entire apartment. During these busy sunsets, Sophie invented a charming little game. She would wait, her little body pulsating with excitement, until Maria had finished mopping the wooden floors with a commercial cleaner. As soon as her mom put away the mop, Sophie would launch herself onto the shiny, still-wet surface, her little feet slipping, her laughter echoing around the high-ceilinged apartment. Maria would look on, her tired eyes lighting up at Sophie's infectious delight, utterly oblivious to the impending danger.

Over time, Sophie's childlike giggles diminished. Instead of her usual energetic self, she became increasingly lethargic after their cleaning game, her rosy cheeks losing warmth and her laughter replaced by weary yawns.

Maria's motherly instincts kicked in. Her vibrant daughter, usually the life of their home, was changing. What was going on with little Sophie?

Maria felt helpless.

Grace, a health-conscious chemist and Maria's college friend, showed up at the door on a chilly Spring evening. Grace watched how Sophie's energy drained following the family's evening cleaning ritual. Grace immediately understood the problem—the fumes from Maria's commercial cleaning products were poisoning Sophie!

Grace, who had spent years promoting natural, eco-friendly alternatives to commercial cleaning agents, explained the impact of the fumes on Sophie's health.

As Grace's words sank in, Maria felt relieved. Her worry transformed into resolve. She threw her old, toxic cleaners in the trash and pledged to use only green options. She now had a tool to revive the once vibrant energy of her little one. She yearned to hear Sophie's carefree laughter filling up their home once again, bouncing off the walls of their snug city apartment.

This chapter will explore the dangers of everyday household cleaning products and chemicals. We'll help you make informed decisions and embrace green alternatives to improve your family and the planet's health. So, let's dive in and unravel the mystery behind the tiny (poisonous) bubbles lurking in our everyday lives.

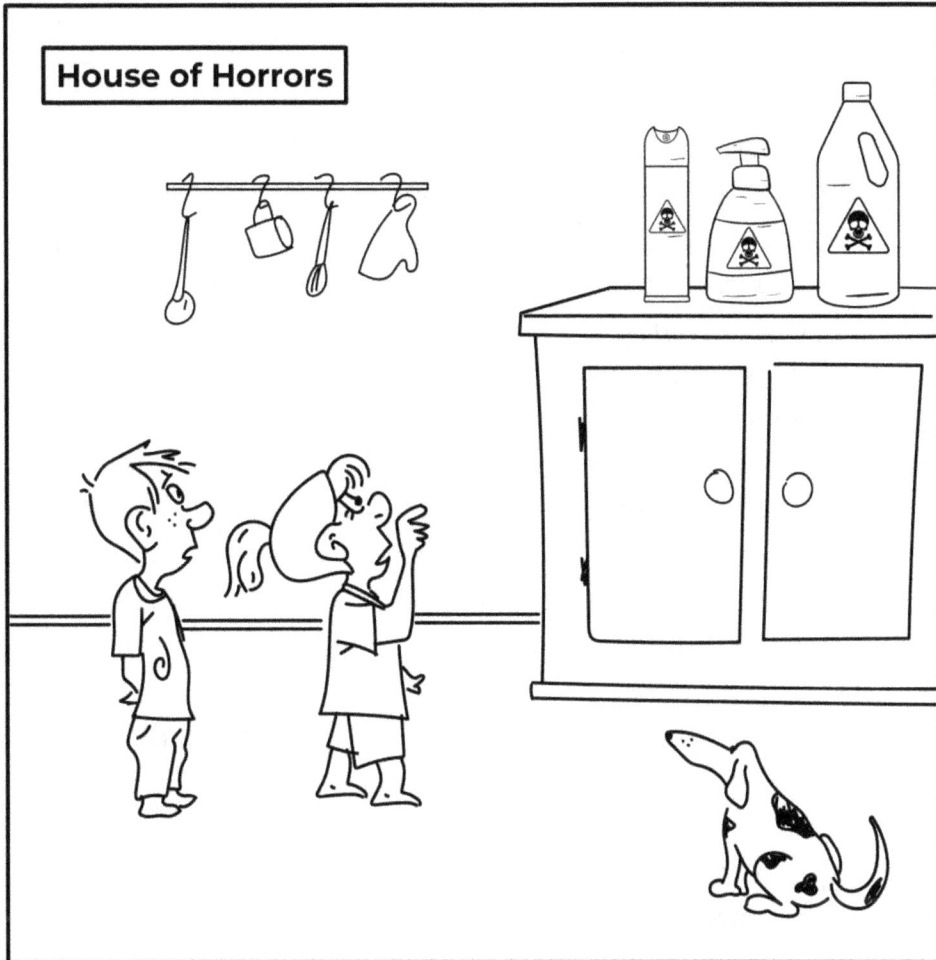

© Dr. Greg, LLC. 2023

What types of common household chemicals and cleaners contain toxic chemicals

As you walk down the cleaning aisle at your local store, you will likely find many products that claim to make your home sparkling clean and germ-free. What you may not realize is that many of these products contain toxic chemicals that can pose significant health risks. Let's take a closer look at some of the most common household cleaners and the potentially harmful ingredients they may contain:

1. All-purpose cleaners: These versatile products are designed to clean various surfaces in your home, but they can contain chemicals such as ammonia, chlorine bleach, and phosphates. Ammonia is a strong irritant that can cause respiratory issues and eye irritation, while chlorine bleach can lead to skin, eye, and respiratory irritation. While they should never be combined, they can still be dangerous even while solo. When released into the environment, phosphates can contribute to water pollution and harm aquatic life.

2. Oven cleaners: Many oven cleaners contain sodium hydroxide, a corrosive chemical that can cause severe burns and respiratory problems if inhaled or ingested. Some oven cleaners include butoxyethanol, a glycol ether solvent associated with liver and kidney damage and reproductive issues.

3. Drain cleaners: These products often contain sodium hydroxide, sulfuric acid, or hydrochloric acid. These highly corrosive chemicals can cause burns, eye damage, and respiratory problems if not handled properly.

4. Toilet bowl cleaners: The chemicals used in toilet bowl cleaners can include chlorine bleach, hydrochloric acid, and sodium lauryl sulfate. Exposure to these substances can lead to skin, eye, and respiratory irritation and damage to the gastrointestinal tract if ingested.

5. Window cleaners: Ammonia and 2-butoxyethanol are common ingredients found in window cleaners. As previously mentioned, ammonia can cause respiratory and eye irritation, while 2-butoxyethanol has been linked to liver and kidney damage and reproductive harm.

6. Air fresheners: Surprisingly, these seemingly innocuous products can contain toxic chemicals such as phthalates, which are used as fragrance carriers, and volatile organic compounds (VOCs), like formaldehyde and benzene. These dangerous solvents can cause respiratory problems,

headaches, and cognitive decline. Some air fresheners may also contain synthetic musks that can disrupt hormone function and have been linked to environmental pollution.

7. Laundry detergents: Conventional laundry detergents often contain surfactants like alkylphenol ethoxylates (APEs) and nonylphenol ethoxylates (NPEs), which can cause skin irritation and appear to disrupt endocrine function in aquatic life when released into the ocean. Some laundry detergents may also contain phosphates, which, as mentioned earlier, can contribute to water pollution.

8. Dishwashing detergents: These products can contain phosphates, chlorine bleach, and surfactants like sodium lauryl sulfate. As previously discussed, these chemicals can cause skin, eye, and respiratory irritation and poison the environment.

9. Floor cleaners: Floor cleaning products may contain VOCs, such as glycol ethers, which have been linked to respiratory issues, liver and kidney damage, and reproductive problems. They may also contain pine oil or phenolic disinfectants, which can cause respiratory and skin irritation and are toxic if inhaled. These substances are what harmed little Sophie.

10. Furniture polish and wood cleaners: These products can contain various harmful chemicals, including VOCs like formaldehyde, toluene, and xylene, which can cause headaches, dizziness, and respiratory issues. Some furniture polishes also contain petroleum distillates, which can be toxic if ingested and cause skin irritation.

11. Carpet cleaners: Carpet cleaning products often contain chemicals such as perchloroethylene, a solvent that can cause dizziness, fatigue, and even liver and kidney damage with long-term exposure. They may also contain naphthalene, a potential carcinogen that can harm the central nervous system and cause breathing problems.

12. Mold and mildew removers: These products frequently contain chlorine bleach, which can cause burns, eye damage, and respiratory irritation if improperly handled.

Maria thought she was doing her daughter a favor by keeping a clean home. Unfortunately, she was unaware of all the toxins lurking in her trusted brands. The takeaway is that many of the ordinary household cleaning products we use daily can contain potentially harmful chemicals that pose risks to our health and the environment.

DR. GREG SAYS

Unhealthy cleaning products and cosmetics

Visit any supermarket. The cleaner aisle is festooned with a dizzying array of sprays, soaps, and personal care products. Shiny bottles promise spotless kitchens, sparkling bathrooms, and the fresh scent of a spring meadow. But behind the colorful labels and enticing fragrances, there's a toxic brew of yuck. A cocktail of synthetic chemicals, some of which could be hazardous to our health.

To bring this point home, let's take a closer look at five common yet potentially harmful substances lurking in your everyday household products:

1. Phthalates: Often found in fragranced household products like air fresheners and dish soap, phthalates are known endocrine disruptors and have been linked to increased risk of breast cancer, early breast development in girls, and reproductive birth defects in males and females.

2. Perchloroethylene or "PERC": A neurotoxin, PERC is a common ingredient in carpet and upholstery cleaners. Health effects may include dizziness, loss of coordination, and other neurologic symptoms.

3. Triclosan: Found in most liquid dishwashing detergents and hand soaps labeled "antibacterial," Triclosan is an aggressive antibacterial agent that can promote the development of drug-resistant bacteria. This ingredient is absolutely unnecessary. Soaps wash away germs! There is no need to add antimicrobial chemicals that seep into our water supply and breed dangerous pathogens.

4. Quarternary Ammonium Compounds, or "QUATS": Used in fabric softener liquids and sheets, QUATS can cause skin and respiratory irritation and have been linked with reproductive harm.

5. 2-Butoxyethanol: A key ingredient in window, kitchen, and multipurpose cleaners, 2-Butoxyethanol can cause sore throats, pulmonary edema, and severe liver and kidney damage.

We need to be aware of these hidden threats in our cleaning cabinets. But we're not doomed to this chemical reality. The first step is to consciously shift toward natural, green alternatives that are as effective, if not more so, without compromising our health.

Now let's turn our gaze toward the cosmetics industry. The situation there is no less troubling. Aside from the fact that many of our favorite lotions, creams, and makeup could contain similar hazardous substances, there's another ethical aspect to this story—animal testing.

Animal testing, sadly, is still very much a reality. Despite bans on animal testing for cosmetics in the UK and the European Union, the practice is still not banned in the United States. According to the FDA, it's often up to individual companies to create their own policies on animal testing. This ambiguity can leave the door open for unnecessary animal suffering.

But what can we, as conscious consumers, do about it?

Look for cruelty-free labels on cosmetics, which indicate that the product and its ingredients haven't been tested on animals. Choose brands that are transparent about their ingredient sourcing and manufacturing practices. Choose household cleaners that are plant-based, biodegradable, and free from synthetic fragrances and dyes.

Thankfully, certain brands seem to take their commitment to health and the environment seriously. Seventh Generation, Method, and Mrs. Meyers use healthier ingredients and never test on animals. You should try them or make your own kid-safe cleaners using lemons, vinegar, and essential oils. It's worth it.

Health risks associated with conventional cleaning products and air fresheners

I know this material is dense, but it is vital. Rather than look at the individual products, let's look at symptoms and illnesses caused by household toxins. You might recognize some of these in your own family. If so, speak to your doctor and consider changing your cleaning routines. Let's examine some of the most common health issues associated with exposure to household chemicals:

1. Respiratory (breathing) problems: Some cleaning products, such as ammonia, chlorine bleach, and VOCs, can cause respiratory irritation and exacerbate existing respiratory issues, such as asthma and allergies. A study published in the *Canadian Medical Association Journal* found that frequent use of household cleaning products could increase the risk of developing childhood asthma. The American Lung Association also warns that certain cleaning supplies can release VOCs, contributing to chronic respiratory issues and allergic reactions. Your cleaner may be to blame if you or a family member has unchecked asthma.

2. Skin irritation and burns: Many cleaning products contain corrosive chemicals, such as sodium hydroxide, hydrochloric acid, and chlorine bleach, which can cause skin irritation, burns, and even permanent damage if you're not careful. Moreover, some products, like laundry and dishwashing detergents, contain surfactants that can cause skin irritation and rashes.

3. Eye irritation and damage: The chemicals in cleaning products can also cause eye irritation and damage. For example, ammonia, chlorine bleach, and acids in drain cleaners can lead to irritation, burns, and even blindness if they come into contact with the eyes.

4. Neurological issues: Exposure to some chemicals in cleaning products, such as perchloroethylene and naphthalene, can result in neurological damage, including dizziness, fatigue, and harm to the central nervous system.

5. Gastrointestinal problems: Ingestion of cleaning products containing corrosive chemicals or petroleum distillates can cause damage to the gastrointestinal tract, leading to nausea, vomiting, diarrhea, and even severe burns in the throat and stomach.

6. Hormonal and endocrine disruption: Certain chemicals, such as phthalates in air fresheners and alkylphenol ethoxylates in laundry detergents, can disrupt hormone

function, leading to reproductive and developmental problems. As discussed earlier, synthetic musks in air fresheners have been shown to disrupt hormone function and have been linked to environmental pollution.

7. Cancer risks: Some cleaning products contain known or suspected carcinogens, such as formaldehyde, benzene, and 1,4-dioxane. You'd be surprised how many substances are allowed in the US but are banned in Europe and around the globe. A study from the University of California, Berkeley, found that traditional and some green cleaning products can release carcinogenic chemicals into the air, highlighting the importance of choosing safer alternatives.

8. Poisoning risks: Accidental ingestion of cleaning products, particularly by children, can lead to poisoning and severe health consequences. Regardless of which cleaners you have at home, you must lock them up and keep them out of reach of kids! According to the American Association of Poison Control Centers, cleaning products are among the most common causes of poisoning in children under six.

9. Environmental impacts: The chemicals in many cleaning products can harm the environment when released into the air or washed down the drain. Phosphates, for example, can contribute to water pollution and distort ecosystems, while surfactants like alkylphenol ethoxylates can disrupt endocrine function in fish and other aquatic animals.

Risks to children and pets

Children and pets are particularly vulnerable to the harmful effects of toxic chemicals found in conventional cleaning products. Their developing immune systems and smaller body sizes make them more susceptible to the negative impacts of these chemicals. Let's examine some of the specific risks that conventional cleaning products pose to children and pets:

1. Accidental ingestion: Young children, in particular, are at risk of accidentally ingesting cleaning products due to their natural curiosity and tendency to explore their environment by putting objects in their mouths. Many household products' colorful, inviting package designs can prove irresistible to young eyes. Ingesting toxic cleaning products can lead to serious health consequences, including poisoning, gastrointestinal problems, and death. Pets, too, may accidentally consume cleaning products, especially if they are stored within their reach or if residues are left on surfaces where they eat or drink. Floors and carpets contain traces of cleaners long after they feel dry, placing cats and dogs at risk after your Spring cleaning.

2. Respiratory issues: As mentioned earlier, exposure to chemicals in cleaning products can cause respiratory problems, exacerbating existing respiratory issues such as asthma and allergies. Children and pets have smaller lung capacities and more delicate lungs, which makes them more vulnerable to the harmful effects of these chemicals.

3. Skin irritation: Children and pets may also be more susceptible to skin irritation caused by exposure to chemicals in cleaning products. Their thinner skin and larger surface area-to-weight ratio make them more prone to absorbing these chemicals, which can cause rashes, burns, and other skin problems.

4. Endocrine disruption: Some cleaning products contain chemicals that can disrupt hormone function, leading to developmental and reproductive problems, including altered puberty. Children and pets, with their developing endocrine systems, are particularly sensitive to these effects.

5. Long-term health risks: Exposure to toxic chemicals in cleaning products during childhood can contribute to long-term health risks, such as cancer, abnormal growth, poor school performance, and learning disabilities. Similarly, pets

may experience long-term health consequences due to exposure to cleaners and solvents.

Green cleaning alternatives and homemade solutions

Green cleaning products from natural, non-toxic, and biodegradable ingredients can effectively clean your home without most of the harmful side effects of conventional chemicals. Here are some ideas for green cleaning alternatives and homemade solutions that you can consider:

1. Vinegar: Vinegar is a versatile, natural cleaner that you can use to clean various surfaces, including glass, countertops, and floors. You can also use vinegar to remove soap scum in the bathroom, clean stainless steel appliances, and remove stains from carpets. Mix equal parts water and white vinegar in a spray bottle for an effective, all-purpose cleaner. Hospitals often use vinegar because it is safe and effective.
2. Baking soda: Baking soda is another natural, surprisingly versatile cleaning agent. It works as a gentle abrasive, making it perfect for scrubbing away grime on sinks, bathtubs, and stovetops. Mix baking soda with a small amount of water to form a paste, then scrub the surface with a sponge or cloth. You can use baking soda to deodorize carpets, garbage cans, and refrigerators.
3. Lemon juice: Lemon juice is a natural, acidic cleaner that can help to dissolve soap scum, remove stains, and freshen surfaces. Lemon juice works to remove hard water stains and polish brass and copper. Mix lemon juice with water in a spray bottle for a fresh-smelling, all-purpose cleaner, or use it undiluted to tackle tough stains on countertops and cutting boards. If you have a lemon tree in your backyard, you're really in luck!

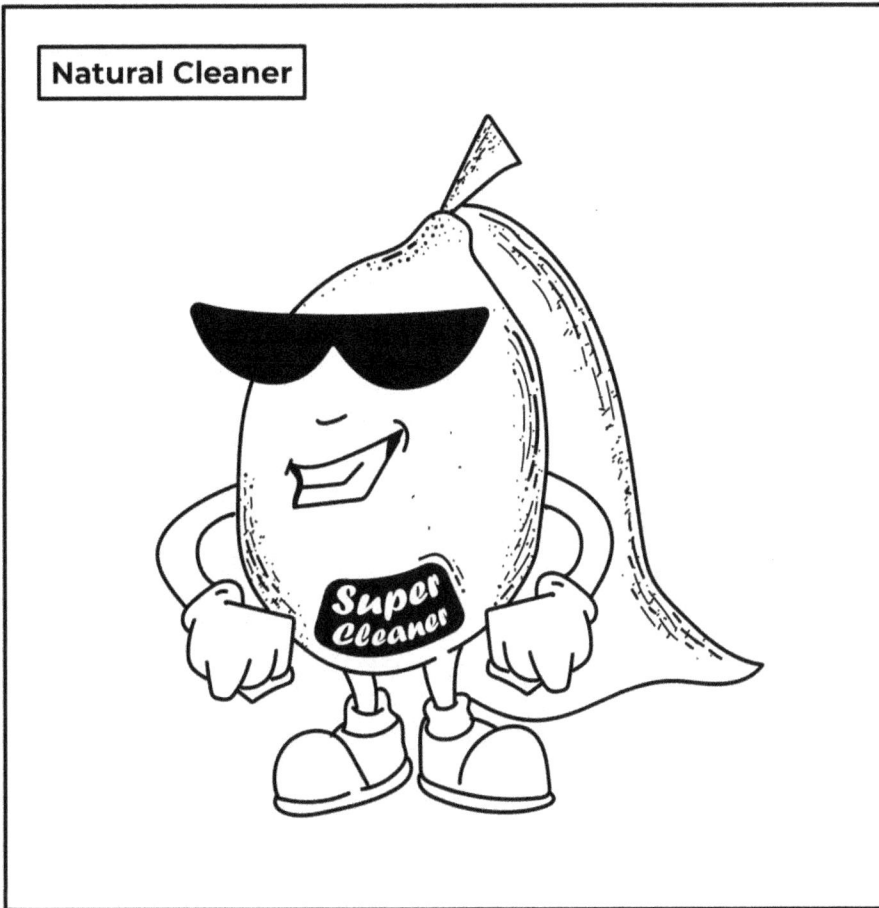

Natural Cleaner

Super Cleaner

4. Castile soap: Castile soap is a plant-based soap used to clean a wide range of surfaces, including floors, countertops, dishes, and laundry. It is biodegradable and gentle on both the environment and your skin. Dilute castile soap with water to create an all-purpose cleaner, or use it directly on a sponge or cloth to clean surfaces.

5. Hydrogen peroxide: Hydrogen peroxide is a natural disinfectant that can kill bacteria, viruses, and mold. It is handy for cleaning cutting boards, disinfecting toothbrushes, and removing stains from clothing and upholstery. Mix equal parts hydrogen peroxide and water in a spray bottle for a safe and effective disinfecting solution.

6. Essential oils: Many essential oils, such as tea tree, lavender, and eucalyptus, have natural antibacterial and antifungal properties that can enhance the cleaning power of your homemade solutions. Add a few drops of your favorite essential oil to a homemade cleaner for a pleasant scent and added cleaning benefits.

7. Microfiber cloths: Instead of using disposable paper towels, consider investing in reusable microfiber cloths. These cloths pick up dirt, dust, and bacteria without harsh chemicals. You can use them wet or dry, and they are machine washable, making them an environmentally friendly and cost-effective alternative to disposable cleaning products.

Benefits of using natural cleaning products in your green home

Switching to natural cleaning products and homemade solutions offers a range of benefits that can improve the overall health and well-being of your family, pets, and the planet. Here are some key advantages of using natural cleaning products in your green home:

1. Improved indoor air quality: As previously discussed, many conventional cleaning products contain volatile organic compounds (VOCs) that can contribute to poor indoor air quality. By choosing natural cleaning products or homemade solutions, you can reduce the number of VOCs released into your home, improving indoor air quality and reducing the risk of respiratory issues and allergies.

2. Reduced health risks: Natural cleaning products are generally free from the toxic chemicals found in conventional cleaning products, which can pose various health risks, including respiratory problems, skin irritation, and long-term health issues such as cancer and neurological damage. The truth is that many of these substances are probably worse than we now understand since it is

impossible to test everything. In other words, there are a lot of unknown unknowns.

3. Safer for children and pets: As we've seen, children and pets are particularly vulnerable to the harmful effects of toxic chemicals in conventional cleaning products.

4. Environmentally friendly: Natural cleaning products are typically biodegradable and made from renewable resources, making them a more sustainable environmental choice. By choosing these products, you can help reduce pollution, conserve resources, and protect aquatic life from the harmful effects of conventional cleaning chemicals. Remember, much of what we use for cleaning will wind up in the oceans. We don't want the dolphins swimming in our solvents.

5. Cost-effective: Many natural cleaning products can be made at home using inexpensive, readily available ingredients, such as vinegar, baking soda, and lemon juice. You'll save money compared with store-bought cleaning products and reduce waste from disposable cleaning supplies, like paper towels.

6. Customizable: When you make your own natural cleaning products, you can customize the ingredients and scents to suit your preferences and needs. This allows you to create personalized cleaning solutions that are effective for your specific cleaning tasks while adding your favorite essential oils for a pleasant fragrance.

7. Reduced chemical exposure for vulnerable populations: Pregnant women, seniors, and people with compromised immune systems are more susceptible to the harmful effects of chemicals found in conventional cleaning products.

8. Supporting eco-friendly companies: By purchasing natural cleaning products from environmentally responsible companies, you're supporting businesses that prioritize sustainability and the health of their customers. This can help to drive demand for greener products and encourage

more companies to adopt eco-friendly practices. Be the change!

9. Increased awareness of ingredients: Switching to natural cleaning products often leads to a greater understanding of the ingredients in the products you use. This can help you make more informed decisions about the products you bring into your home, ensuring a healthier and safer living environment. Plus, reading labels will make you fun and interesting at parties.

10. Community impact: When you use natural cleaning products, you contribute to a larger movement of individuals making environmentally conscious choices. This collective effort can help reduce harmful chemicals' overall impact on our communities and the environment.

I sincerely hope you're enjoying the book so far. If you find the book helpful, please take a moment and share *Dr. Greg's Green Home Makeover* with a friend and write an honest 5-star review online. Thank you for helping to spread the word and build a green community!

CHAPTER 5

Poison In Purple:

Paints and Adhesives

Ever since she was a little girl, Penny has had a deep love for colors. It didn't matter if it was the bright, buttery yellow of sunflowers or the soothing, cool aquamarine of the ocean, every hue had a story to tell, and Penny loved to listen. Now, as an adult, her life was as vibrant as her favorite rainbow mural, filled with passion for her job as an interior designer and her side gig: running a small, bustling shelter for puppies.

Among the playful pooches in "The Pup Palette," Waffles, a honey-coated Golden Retriever, held a special place in Penny's heart. Waffles flashed his zest for life, zipping around the lime green of the main play area, his favorite space in the shelter. He would spend his days bouncing in the room, the lively color fueling his endless games of chase and tug-of-war.

One day, Penny was adding another coat of lime green to the playroom walls when she felt a change. Her sudden, unexpected cough shattered the silence. Penny's hacking smashed the room's peace. She glanced around to find Waffles, her usually playful companion, mirroring her symptoms. His eyes, normally full of energy, clouded with discomfort. The pungent, overwhelming aroma of the fresh paint filled the room, making the air feel dense and suffocating.

Worried about her beloved pups, Penny threw open the windows and rushed everyone outside.

She plunged into a deep dive into the world of paints and read about Volatile Organic Compounds (VOCs). She learned about the harmful gases these compounds released into the air and the potential impact on health. This newfound knowledge felt like a punch in the stomach, and guilt washed over her. Were her colors poisoning her beloved pups?

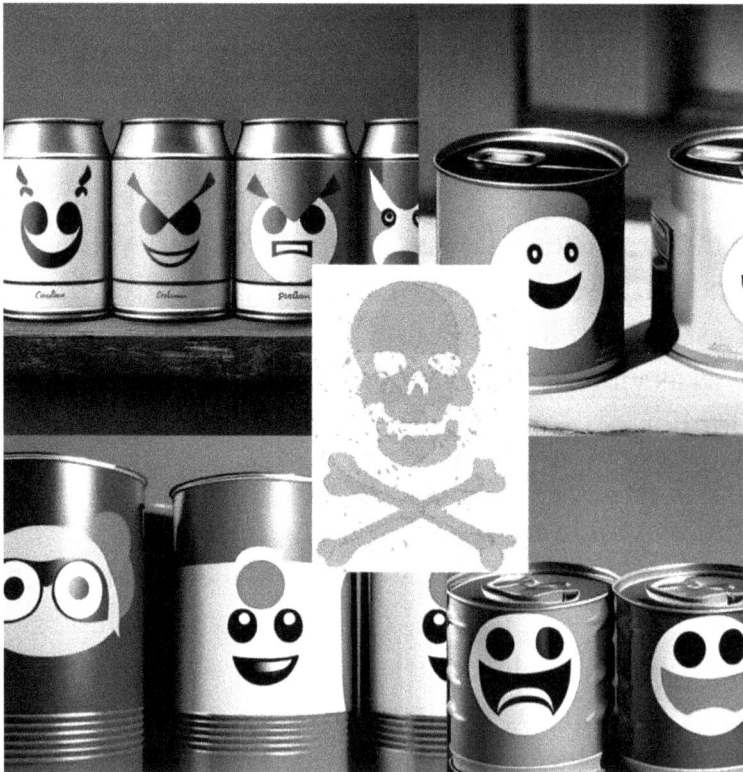

Penny resolved to change. She couldn't bear the thought of her passion causing harm to Waffles and the other furballs in her shelter. Determined to maintain the colorful spirit of the facility while ensuring its safety, she set out on a mission to find a better solution.

Penny discovered paints and adhesives with low or no VOCs. She transformed "The Pup Palette," replacing the potentially harmful paints with safer alternatives. As she applied the final brushstroke to the lime green play area, she could almost feel the room breathe easier. Waffles seemed to sense it, too, his tail wagging with zeal.

With Waffles hopping around in the newly revitalized, safer space, Penny worked with all her interior design clients to help them transition to safer, greener products. After all, color should bring the world joy, not harm.

Volatile Organic Compounds (VOCs) are a diverse group of organic chemicals that easily evaporate at room temperature, releasing potentially harmful gases into the air. Found in a wide range of household and building products, VOCs can significantly impact indoor air quality and contribute to numerous illnesses.

Common sources of VOCs in homes and buildings include paints, solvents, adhesives, sealants, carpets, and wood products. VOCs spew into the air when we use or store these products indoors, generating potentially toxic levels in our homes.

Paints are a major source of VOCs in homes and buildings. Traditional solvent-based paints, also known as oil-based or alkyd paints, often contain high levels of VOCs that evaporate as the paint dries. The solvents used in these paints are typically derived from petroleum and are responsible for the strong odors associated with fresh paint. In contrast, water-based or latex paints contain lower levels of VOCs but may still emit harmful compounds during the drying process.

VOCs are typically used as solvents to help the paint dry faster, spread more evenly, and adhere better to surfaces. In sealants and adhesives, VOCs serve as the "carrier, " allowing the product to flow and bond to different materials. As these products dry or cure, they leach VOCs into the air, contributing to indoor air pollution.

Adhesives and sealants used in construction and renovation projects can also release VOCs into the air. These products often contain solvents that help maintain the adhesive or sealant in a liquid state before application, then evaporate during curing. Examples of adhesives and sealants with high VOC content include those used for attaching wall coverings, flooring materials, countertops, and caulks and glues.

Flooring materials can be another significant source of VOCs in homes and buildings. Carpets, for instance, can emit VOCs from the synthetic fibers, adhesives, and backing materials used in their construction. Some engineered wood products, such as plywood, particleboard, and medium-density fiberboard (MDF), contain formaldehyde-based resins that release VOCs over time.

Household cleaning products, air fresheners, and even some personal care items can contribute to indoor VOC levels. Many of these products contain fragrances or solvents that emit VOCs when used or stored in the home. It's important to note that "natural" or "organic" products may still contain VOCs, as the term "organic" refers to the chemical structure or sourcing of these compounds and not necessarily their safety.

In addition to these familiar sources, VOCs can off-gas from other household items and building materials, such as upholstered furniture, draperies, and insulation. Tobacco smoke (yuck!), wood-burning stoves, and certain cooking appliances increase indoor VOC levels.

One popular misconception about VOCs is that they are only found in synthetic or chemical-based products. However, relatively natural materials can also emit VOCs. For example, wood products like plywood and particleboard often release formaldehyde, a harmful VOC. Some essential oils, which many folks assume are natural and safe, can emit VOCs when diffused in the air.

With so many potential sources of VOCs in our homes and buildings, it's crucial to understand the health risks associated with exposure to these compounds and take steps to weed these buggers out.

In the next section, we'll delve deeper into the health risks associated with VOC exposure and discuss ways to minimize these risks during home renovations and remodeling projects.

Health risks

VOCs can pose significant health risks, particularly at high indoor concentrations. These risks can range from short-term effects, such as irritation of the eyes, nose, and throat, to more severe long-term consequences, like damage to the liver, kidneys, and central nervous system. Some VOCs, like benzene and formaldehyde, are classified as carcinogens and can increase cancer risk.

One common misconception is that only people with chemical sensitivities or allergies are at risk of health issues due to VOC exposure. While these individuals may be more susceptible, everyone can suffer from VOCs, depending on the concentration and duration of exposure.

Short-term exposure to high levels of VOCs can lead to immediate health effects, including headaches, dizziness, and nausea. These symptoms are collectively called "sick building syndrome" or "building-related illness." People who work in offices with poor ventilation or spend long hours in newly painted or remodeled spaces are particularly at risk of experiencing these problems.

Long-term exposure to VOCs can have more severe health consequences. Studies have linked chronic exposure to VOCs with an increased risk of asthma, allergies, and other respiratory disorders. Additionally, research has suggested that exposure to VOCs during critical periods of development, such as during pregnancy or early childhood, can have lasting effects on children's cognitive, behavioral, and motor development (see below). Furthermore, chronic exposure to certain VOCs, like formaldehyde, has been associated with an increased risk of cancer.

It's important to note that not all VOCs are created equal. Different compounds have varying toxicity levels and health effects. For example, some VOCs, like acetone, are relatively low in toxicity and pose minimal health risks. In contrast, others, like benzene, are highly toxic and can cause serious health problems even at low concentrations.

Considering the potential health risks associated with VOC exposure, it's crucial to reduce these compounds' presence in our homes and buildings. One effective way to do this is by choosing low-VOC or zero-VOC products during home renovations and remodeling projects (see below).

Children, pets, the elderly, and pregnant women are at the highest risk

Specific populations are particularly vulnerable to the harmful effects of VOCs. Children, pets, the elderly, and pregnant women are among those who face the highest risk due to their unique physiological characteristics and behaviors.

Children are especially susceptible to the effects of VOCs for several reasons. First, their respiratory rates and metabolism are higher than adults', meaning they inhale more air relative to their body weight and, consequently, a higher concentration of VOCs. Additionally, children's developing bodies and immune systems make them more vulnerable to the toxic effects of these chemicals. VOC exposure during critical developmental periods can lead to long-lasting health issues, including behavioral and motor deficits.

Exposure to VOCs can harm children's cognitive development. According to a study published in *Environment International*, there is an association between higher levels of VOC exposure in childhood and decreased mental function, affecting areas such as attention, memory, and reasoning. Children exposed to high levels of VOCs in their homes have shown a decrease in their IQ scores. Long-term exposure can also lead to severe health issues such as asthma, allergies, and other respiratory disorders.

Chronic exposure to VOCs can also lead to the development of childhood leukemia and lymphomas. According to a report by the Minnesota Department of Health, home environments with elevated levels of VOCs, such as benzene, are associated with an increased risk of these types of cancers in children.

Pets, like children, are at increased risk due to their smaller size and faster metabolism. They are also more likely to be in close contact with surfaces and materials that emit VOCs, such as carpets, upholstery, and flooring. This close contact can lead to toxic exposure.

VOCs have been linked to various respiratory issues in pets, including asthma and bronchitis. Since pets often spend more time indoors and near the ground where VOC concentrations can be higher, their exposure levels can be substantial. One study published in the *Journal of Veterinary Medical Science* has shown a significant association between VOC exposure and respiratory diseases in dogs. Long-term exposure can lead to chronic respiratory illnesses, severely affecting their quality of life.

VOCs can also damage a pet's liver, kidney, and central nervous system. The metabolism of many VOCs occurs in the liver and kidneys, and high levels of exposure can overwhelm these organs, leading to toxicity. The damage may not be immediate and could manifest over time with continued exposure. One study reported in *Environmental Science and Pollution Research International* showed that pets exposed to high levels of VOCs had higher rates of liver and kidney diseases.

I can speak from experience on this one. Other than walking outdoors or horsing around with a tennis ball, my pup spends most of her day lying on the carpet, often with her head hidden underneath the couch. It's a good gig! Except, of course, her sensitive lungs are inhaling all the nasty gasses and fumes leaking out of our flooring. Am I unknowingly poisoning her?

Elderly individuals may face a heightened risk from VOC exposure because their immune systems are often weaker, making them more susceptible to infections and diseases. Additionally, pre-existing health conditions, such as respiratory or cardiovascular diseases, can be exacerbated by VOC exposure.

Pregnant women are another high-risk group for VOC exposure. VOCs can cross the placenta, potentially affecting fetal development and increasing the risk of birth defects or developmental disorders.

A study in the *International Journal of Environmental Research and Public Health* discovered that pregnant women with high exposure to VOCs had significantly higher risks of delivering preterm babies. In addition, there was an increase in the likelihood of low birth weight in newborns exposed to VOCs in utero.

Prenatal exposure to certain VOCs may also impact neurodevelopment in fetuses, potentially leading to neurobehavioral problems in childhood. A study published by the National Center for Biotechnology Information indicates a significant association between prenatal VOC exposure and impairments in areas such as attention span, memory, and language development.

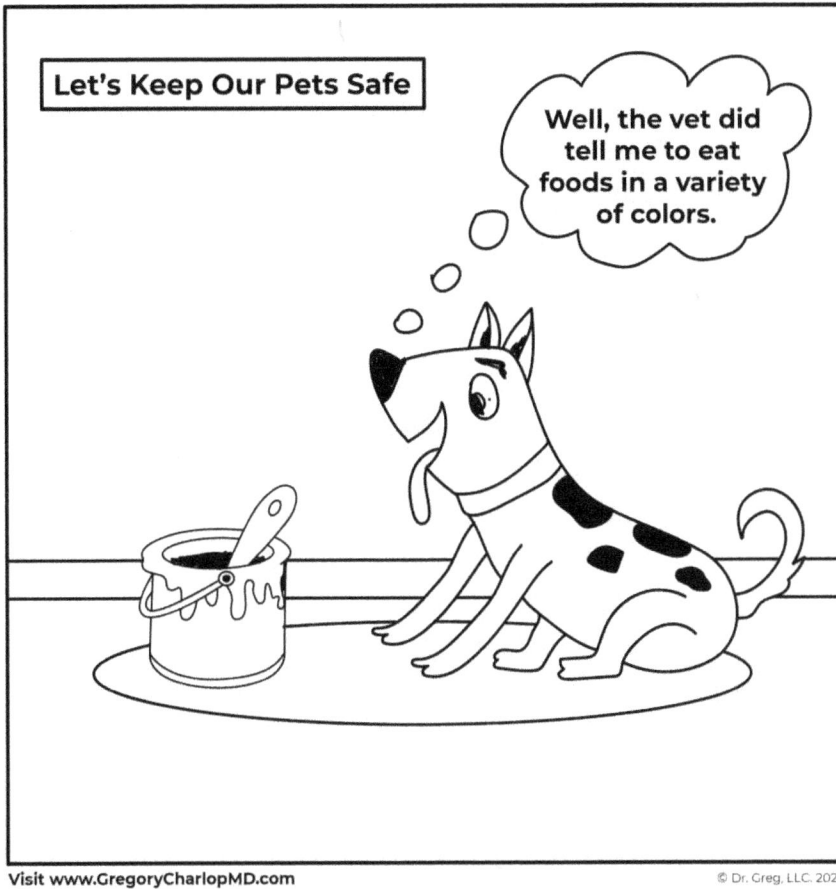

Given the heightened vulnerability of these populations, it's essential to prioritize reducing VOC exposure, particularly in homes and environments where they spend significant amounts of time. It's time to use low-VOC or zero-VOC products during home renovations and remodeling projects.

Choosing low-VOC and zero-VOC products for your remodel

When planning a green home remodel, one of the most effective ways to protect the health of your family and the environment is by choosing low-VOC or zero-VOC products. These products have significantly lower levels of harmful VOCs than traditional building materials and can help maintain healthier indoor air.

1. Paints: Low-VOC and zero-VOC paints are now widely available, offering a healthier alternative to conventional products that emit high levels of VOCs. These eco-friendly paints use water as the primary solvent instead of petroleum-based products, reducing the emission of harmful VOCs during drying. It's important to note that zero-VOC paints may still contain trace amounts of VOCs, but the levels are significantly lower than in traditional alternatives.

2. Adhesives and Sealants: Low-VOC adhesives and sealants minimize the release of VOCs during application and curing. These products use water-based or low-VOC solvents, providing a safer and more environmentally friendly option for your kitchen and bathroom.

3. Flooring: Some types of flooring, such as carpeting and engineered wood, can emit massive amounts of VOCs, particularly during installation. Choose flooring materials certified as low-VOC or zero-VOC to reduce VOC exposure, such as solid hardwood, bamboo, or cork. Additionally, look for products with third-party certifications like FloorScore® or GreenGuard, which ensure that the materials meet stringent standards for emissions. Side note, bamboo flooring looks awesome!

4. Cabinetry and Wood Products: As mentioned earlier, wood products like plywood and particleboard can release formaldehyde, a harmful VOC. Choose solid wood cabinetry or products made from formaldehyde-free alternatives like medium-density fiberboard (MDF) or wheatboard to minimize exposure. Look for products that have been certified by organizations like the Composite Panel Association or the California Air Resources Board, which set strict standards for formaldehyde emissions in wood products.

When selecting low-VOC and zero-VOC products for your remodel, read product labels carefully and verify the claims made by manufacturers. Some products may be marketed as "green" or "eco-friendly" without meeting the criteria for low-VOC emissions. Third-party certifications, such as GreenGuard, Green Seal®, or the Environmental Protection Agency's (EPA) Indoor airPLUS program, can help you identify products that meet low-VOC or zero-VOC standards. I'm thankful I switched to healthier rugs and furniture, so my kids and pup can breathe a little easier.

Special circumstances: hospitals, homes for seniors, and nurseries

In environments like hospitals, retirement homes, and nurseries, where vulnerable populations spend a significant amount of time, it's even more crucial to prioritize using low-VOC and zero-VOC products in building and renovation projects. These settings require special attention to indoor air quality to protect the health and well-being of patients, residents, and staff.

In hospitals, poor indoor air quality can exacerbate existing health conditions and compromise the recovery of patients, especially those with respiratory or immune system issues. Using low-VOC and zero-VOC products in hospital renovations can help prevent complications and promote faster healing.

Reducing VOC exposure is essential in homes for older people, where residents often have weakened immune systems and pre-existing health conditions. These facilities can provide residents with a safer and healthier environment by choosing low-VOC and zero-VOC cabinets, flooring, and paint. Plus, they're a great selling point for potential new tenants!

Nurseries and childcare facilities also need to prioritize indoor air quality due to the heightened vulnerability of young children to VOC exposure. Using low-VOC and zero-VOC products in these settings can help protect children's developing bodies and minds, minimizing the risk of developmental issues related to VOC exposure.

We must prioritize pure, breathable air in all of these unique locations. Designers should prioritize windows and doors to draw in fresh outdoor air, HVAC systems to increase air circulation, indoor plants, and filters to remove impurities.

CHAPTER 6

Free Money:
A Home Energy Audit

In the quiet, unsuspecting neighborhood of Spruce Greens, a homeowner named Jack was as practical as he was cunning. Jack's dream was simple: an epic getaway to the Caribbean with his family. However, each time he tried to save up for this much-desired vacation, he was thwarted by a formidable adversary - his own home.

No matter how diligently Jack scrimped and saved, his utility bills loomed large, holding his vacation dreams hostage. Jack felt the chilling drafts from his creaky old windows, heard the incessant hum of his ancient refrigerator, and cursed the sweltering heat of his home during the summer months. All these energy-guzzling culprits seemed to conspire against him, bleeding his savings dry and foiling his grand vacation plans. Jack vowed to wage war on this energy-draining nemesis, and it was then that he discovered the secret weapon of home energy audits.

Jack was determined to outsmart these energy thieves. He became intimately familiar with the intricacies of insulation, the secrets of air sealing, and the fine art of upgrading appliances. He realized that he needed to become the ultimate energy efficiency operative to defeat his unseen adversaries and restore the balance of power in his home.

As Jack embarked on his mission to reclaim his long-awaited Caribbean dream vacation, he couldn't help but feel a sense of exhilaration. Little did he know, his journey into the realm of energy audits would save his vacation dreams and transform his home into a fortress of efficiency and comfort.

Imagine waking up one morning and discovering a treasure trove of free money hidden under your mattress. Sounds too good to be true, right? Well, that's the kind of surprise you could experience when you conduct a home energy audit. You might not find literal piles of cash, but the potential energy and cost savings you'll uncover will be nearly as rewarding.

So, what exactly is a home energy audit? Simply put, it's a comprehensive assessment of your home's energy use and efficiency. The goal is to identify ways to reduce energy consumption, improve the comfort of your living space, and save money on utility bills—all while contributing to a healthier planet. You'll love the benefits of a more energy-efficient home: lower energy costs, reduced environmental impact, and a cozier living environment. And as a doctor, I can assure you that a greener home can improve your family's physical and mental health.

Conducting a home energy audit is like giving your home a thorough check-up. You'll examine the building envelope (the physical barriers that separate the indoors from the outdoors), heating and cooling systems, appliances, lighting, and water usage. By analyzing these elements, you can pinpoint areas where you're wasting energy, identify opportunities for improvement, and prioritize projects with the greatest impact on your home's energy efficiency and comfort.

The benefits of a home energy audit are undeniable. According to ENERGY STAR (a joint program from the US Environmental Protection Agency and Department of Energy that helps consumers identify energy-efficient products and services), a typical American household spends about $2,200 a year on energy bills. Energy-efficient improvements identified in an audit can save a substantial fraction of those costs. That's hundreds of dollars you can save annually.

For the record, those auditors must not live in my house; my charges seem much higher!

In addition to the financial and environmental benefits, a home energy audit can also improve your family's health and well-being. Energy-efficient homes have better indoor air quality, which can help reduce respiratory issues like asthma and allergies. They maintain a more consistent temperature, reducing the risk of mold and mildew growth. In short, a home energy audit is a simple but powerful tool to help you create a healthier, greener, and more cost-effective living space.

Now that we've established the importance of a home energy audit, it's time to dive into the two main approaches: Do-It-Yourself (DIY) and professional audits. In the next section, we'll explore the differences between these two methods and help you decide which meets your needs.

What's the Difference Between a DIY and a Professional Audit?

Both approaches have pros and cons, and the choice ultimately comes down to your individual needs, budget, and comfort level with home improvement tasks.

A DIY home energy audit is exactly what it sounds like, a self-guided assessment of your home's energy use and efficiency. This approach can be appealing because it's low-cost and allows you to work at your own pace. To perform a DIY audit, you'll need to examine your insulation, air sealing, heating and cooling systems, lighting, and appliances, to identify potential energy-saving opportunities. You can find numerous resources online, including step-by-step guides and checklists, to help you conduct a thorough and accurate assessment.

The DIY approach has its advantages, but it's essential to recognize that it may not be as comprehensive as a professional audit. While you can identify some energy-saving opportunities, you could miss more complex or hidden issues that a trained professional could detect. Additionally, conducting a DIY audit requires some familiarity with home construction, energy systems, and safety precautions, so it's not for everyone.

A professional home energy audit, on the other hand, involves hiring a certified energy auditor or contractor to evaluate your home's energy efficiency. These professionals have the training, experience, and specialized tools to thoroughly and accurately assess your home's energy use. They can also help you prioritize and implement energy-saving improvements and connect you with financial incentives or rebates for certain projects.

The primary downside of a professional audit is the cost. While prices can vary depending on your location and the size of your home, a professional audit typically costs between $300 and $500. Thankfully, the energy savings you'll uncover can often offset the upfront cost of the audit. They may also be tax deductible.

Which approach is right for you? If you're comfortable with home improvement tasks and are primarily interested in identifying simple, low-cost energy-saving opportunities, a DIY audit might be the way to go (or at least to begin the process). You might even enjoy the treasure hunt. However, a professional audit is likely better if you seek a more comprehensive assessment and guidance on implementing improvements. Ultimately, the decision comes down to your individual needs and preferences, but whichever route you choose, you'll take a decisive step toward a greener, more energy-efficient home.

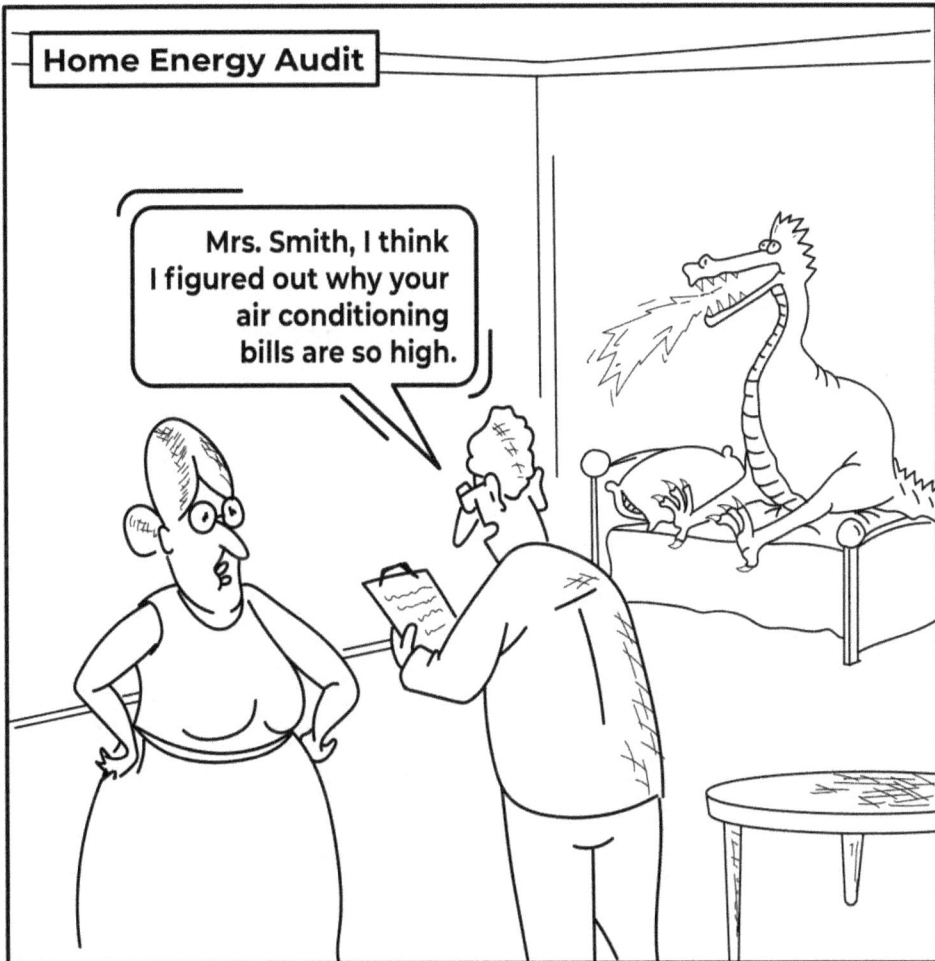

DR. GREG SAYS

Healthy home audits

For select individuals and businesses, my team and I perform healthy home audits, a novel practice far beyond traditional home inspections. People contact us to ensure their kids and pets are safe at home. It is not merely about ticking checkboxes on safety standards or structural stability. Instead, we focus on the broader scope of wellness—health, environmental sustainability, and productivity within your living and working spaces.

Our intention is not to judge but to provide personalized advice that could turn your homes and offices into spaces that nurture the inhabitants and the environment. To optimize your health and environmental sustainability, we consider an array of often overlooked factors.

We begin our process with a thorough understanding of your needs and aspirations for remodeling. We are not here to impose a one-size-fits-all solution but rather to tailor a solution to your unique situation and goals. Our experience enables us to craft a clear and specific roadmap to a healthier and more productive home.

Let's take air quality, for instance. Clean air can reduce your family's danger from allergies, asthma, and infectious diseases. When your children breathe unhealthy air, they're at risk for problems at school and a lifetime of chronic disease. Therefore, we evaluate the ventilation and filtration systems and provide specific suggestions that range from using advanced air purifiers to incorporating natural elements like houseplants that detoxify the air.

The powerful connection between light, mood, and productivity is central to our approach. We help you optimize light in your living spaces—through optimal window placement, intelligent light fixtures, and the strategic use of artificial lights. It's about creating a bright, cheerful atmosphere that stimulates alertness and energy in the morning for productive work and a calm, sleep-promoting environment at dusk.

As animal lovers, we offer advice on pet-friendly landscaping, using plants that are non-toxic to animals, and designing outdoor spaces that are secure and enjoyable for your furry friends. We ensure your companions are safe in and around your home.

As part of our commitment to sustainability, we guide you in choosing energy-efficient appliances, superior insulation, and other features that reduce your carbon footprint. You'll save on utility bills and protect the planet for future generations.

If you want your home or business considered for our in-person or FaceTime healthy home audit, please reach out at www.GregoryCharlopMD.com. Since our in-person availability is limited, we hope this book will help you, our readers, conduct your own health home audits!

A 12-Step DIY Green Home Audit

Congratulations if you've decided to embark on a DIY home energy audit! You're taking a significant step toward a greener, more cost-effective, and healthier home. To help guide you through the process, we've compiled a 12-step DIY green home audit checklist. These steps help you evaluate your home's energy and water efficiency and identify areas where you can spruce things up. So, grab your flashlight, and let's get started!

1. Check insulation levels: Insulation is essential for maintaining a comfortable indoor temperature and minimizing energy loss through the building envelope. Start by examining your attic, walls, and basement or crawlspace insulation. Look for cracks, gaps, or inconsistencies, and ensure the insulation is up to the recommended levels for your climate.

2. Seal air leaks: Air leaks can be a significant source of energy waste, letting warm or cool air escape your home and forcing your HVAC system to work harder. Inspect windows, doors, skylights, and other potential sources of drafts (such as electrical outlets and baseboards) for air leaks. You can

use a lit incense stick to help detect drafts: if the smoke wavers or is blown away, you've found an air leak. Seal any gaps with weatherstripping, caulk, or expandable foam.

3. Inspect heating and cooling systems: Your HVAC (heating, ventilation, and air conditioning) system is likely one of the largest energy consumers in your home. To ensure it's running efficiently, start by examining the condition of your furnace or heat pump, air conditioner or evaporative cooler, and ductwork. Check for any obvious issues, such as dirty filters, blocked vents, or damaged ducts. I'm telling you, check those filters! I've ruined a furnace with a nasty, clogged filter I left in for too long. Make sure that your thermostat is functioning correctly, and consider upgrading to a programmable or smart thermostat, which can help optimize your heating and cooling schedule for maximum efficiency. Regular maintenance is crucial for the longevity and performance of your HVAC system. Proper care can improve your system's efficiency and extend its lifespan, saving you money in the long run. Schedule annual tune-ups with a professional technician who can inspect, clean, and service your equipment, identify potential problems, and recommend any necessary repairs or upgrades. By the way, many home warranty companies will provide a technician to inspect your HVAC system (and filter!) at a low cost.

4. Assess lighting: Swap out incandescent bulbs with more energy-efficient options like compact fluorescent lamps (CFLs) or light-emitting diode (LED) bulbs. Consider using dimmer switches, timers, or motion sensors to reduce energy consumption.

5. Evaluate appliances: Older appliances can be greedy energy hogs. Check the age and efficiency of your refrigerator, dishwasher, washing machine, and dryer. If they're outdated, consider upgrading to ENERGY STAR-certified models, which use significantly less energy and water.

6. Check for vampire power: Many electronics and appliances continue to draw power even when turned off or not in use, a phenomenon known as "vampire power" or "standby power." This can add up over time and contribute to higher energy bills. Examples of devices that draw standby power include televisions, computers, gaming consoles, phone chargers, and even coffee makers. To tackle vampire power, first, identify which devices in your home might be culprits. Then, consider using power strips with built-in switches, smart plugs, or timer switches to cut off power when these devices are not in use. Another strategy is to group devices typically used together, like a TV and a gaming console, on the same power strip. This way, you can turn off multiple devices simultaneously when you're done using them.

7. Examine water heater efficiency: Inspect your water heater for any signs of wear or inefficiency, such as corrosion or leaks. Consider insulating the tank and hot water pipes to reduce heat loss and improve efficiency.

8. Evaluate window efficiency: Windows can be a significant source of heat loss in the winter and heat gain in the summer. Inspect your windows for drafts, damaged seals, or single-pane construction. Consider upgrading to energy-efficient double or triple-pane windows or installing window film or shades to help reduce heat transfer.

9. Renewable energy options: As you improve your home's energy efficiency, remember the potential benefits of renewable energy sources like solar panels or wind turbines. Research the feasibility of installing these systems in your area and the financial incentives that might be available.

Now that we've covered the energy portion of your audit, let's move on to water efficiency:

10. Inspect faucets, showerheads, and toilets: Leaky faucets, inefficient showerheads, and older toilets can waste a significant amount of water, leading to higher utility bills and

water shortages. Start by checking all the faucets in your home for leaks, paying close attention to the spout and the handles. A single dripping tap can waste more than 3,000 gallons of water annually, so fixing leaks promptly is essential. Regarding showerheads, evaluate the flow rate and consider upgrading to a low-flow or WaterSense-labeled model, which can use up to 40% less water than a standard showerhead. Check toilets for leaks around the base or from the tank into the bowl. You can do this by adding a few drops of food coloring to the tank and waiting to see if the color appears in the bowl. If you have an older toilet, consider upgrading to a high-efficiency or dual-flush model, which can use up to 60% less water than a traditional toilet. Addressing these water-wasting fixtures can significantly reduce your home's water consumption and save money on your water bill.

11. Examine outdoor water use: Outdoor water use, such as landscaping and irrigation, can account for a substantial portion of your home's water consumption. Inspect your sprinkler system for leaks and misaligned or broken sprinkler heads, and ensure that you water only during the early morning or late evening to minimize evaporation. Consider implementing drought-tolerant landscaping or rain barrels to collect water for outdoor use.

12. Evaluate water-using appliances: Examine your water heater and other appliances, like dishwashers and washing machines. Check for leaks and consider upgrading to water-efficient models if they're outdated. Remember to run your clothes washer only when full to maximize efficiency.

And there you have it—a 12-step DIY green home audit to help you assess your home's energy and water efficiency. By following these steps, you'll be well on your way to uncovering potential energy and water-saving opportunities that can save you money and contribute to a healthier, more environmentally-friendly home. Remember, small changes generate significant savings over time, so don't be afraid to start with the low-hanging fruit and work your way up to more extensive improvements.

As you tackle your DIY audit, remember that you may still benefit from a professional assessment down the road, especially if you encounter complex issues or require expert guidance. Whichever path you choose, the important thing is that you're taking proactive steps to create a greener, more efficient, and healthier home for yourself and your loved ones.

With all the dough you'll save, you can gift several copies of this book to friends and family to show them how much you care!

CHAPTER 7

Windows and Doors:
From Panes to Gains

Sarah Jenkins was always one for a good challenge, and the eccentric, century-old house she'd recently acquired fit the bill. It was the kind of house with its own personality—creaky floorboards that talked back, wallpaper that whispered stories from the past, and windows and doors that sighed with every gust of wind. It was charming, her sister said, but as the winter started to set in, the house's quirks were beginning to feel less cute and more... chilly.

One particularly frosty Boston evening, Sarah sat huddled in her favorite armchair, a stack of unopened utility bills glaring at her from the coffee table. She was swathed in sweaters and wrapped in blankets, but still, the cold was relentless, seeping in through the single-pane windows and the gaps around the doors. She could almost hear the house chuckling at her futile attempts to stay warm.

She was sick of it.

What if she could turn the tables on the old house? What if she could make it work with her instead of against her? With a healthy mix of desperation and resolve, she reached for her laptop and began researching energy-efficient windows and doors. The more she read, the more she realized this was her answer. Not only could she make the house warmer and more comfortable, but she could also decrease her utility bills and reduce her carbon footprint. Take that, utility bills!

But, like any good challenge, it wouldn't be easy. Energy-efficient windows and doors weren't cheap, and the choices were overwhelming. The options seemed endless: single, double, and triple-paned windows, low-E coatings, and various door materials. But Sarah, always a fan of a good mystery, was excited to unravel the complexities.

And so, our heroine embarked on a new quest: to turn her vintage, drafty house into a green, energy-efficient haven. And as she navigated the world of U-values, SHGC, and Energy Star ratings, she found a sense of purpose and excitement she hadn't felt in a long time.

As this chapter unfolds, we'll accompany Sarah on her journey, exploring the benefits and challenges of energy-efficient windows and doors. We'll decipher the jargon, discuss the different types and their benefits, and shed light on potential energy and cost savings, along with available federal tax credits and programs. So, let's get this show on the road!

When to change your windows and doors

When dealing with an old furnace, screaming toddlers, and an out-of-control work schedule, it's easy to overlook your windows and doors. That's a mistake. There are several hints that it may be time to replace your windows and doors, and being aware of these signs can help you make informed decisions about upgrades.

When you notice drafts or air leaks around the frames, it's time to replace your windows. Drafty windows dramatically impact your home's energy efficiency and temperature, allowing cold air to enter and warm air to escape. You really shouldn't feel drafts by closed windows.

You need to hit the hardware store if you have single-pane windows. Single-pane windows are less energy-efficient than double or triple-pane options, blowing up your utility bills.

Condensation between the panes of glass in double or triple-pane windows can also signal that it's time for a change. This condensation indicates that the window's seal has failed, reducing its insulating properties and energy efficiency.

Similarly, when it comes to doors, if you notice drafts, warping, or difficulty opening and closing, these issues may be signs that it's time for an upgrade.

Finally, consider the age and overall condition of your windows and doors. Windows and doors have a lifespan, and their energy efficiency and performance can decrease as they age. If your windows or doors show signs of wear, such as peeling paint, rot, or rust, it may be time for a replacement.

How to read the label: A Brief explanation of U rating, climate zones, and other factors on the label

Here's the confusing stuff. Let's look at the various labels and rating schemes to help you make informed decisions. The U rating, climate zones, and heat coefficients will guide you toward the right products for your location and budget.

In the simplest terms, the U-factor (or U-rating) measures the rate at which heat is lost through a window or a door. It's like the window's report card for insulation—a lower number means it's doing a better job keeping the heat in (or out, depending on the season).

The U-factor typically ranges from 0.25 to 1.25 and is measured in BTU/h·ft²·°F. So, when considering a window or door, remember this rule of thumb: the lower the U-factor, the better the insulation.

The optimal U-factor for your windows and doors can vary depending on location. For instance, in a colder city like Minneapolis or Chicago, you'd want windows with a lower U-factor, ideally below 0.30, to prevent heat loss during those frigid winters. On the other hand, if you're in a warmer city like Miami or Houston, a higher U-factor works fine, as cooling rather than heating is the primary concern. Still, energy-efficient windows with low U-factors can also help keep your home cool by reducing the heat that enters from the outside, making them a smart choice regardless of your local climate.

Choosing the right U-factor is about more than just comfort. It can also have a significant impact on your energy bills. According to Energy Star, replacing old windows with energy-efficient ones can save you hundreds of dollars per year, depending on your location. Moreover, you may also be eligible for federal tax credits or other incentives for improving your home's energy efficiency. Now you see why Sarah was so enthusiastic about her new windows!

The Solar Heat Gain Coefficient, or SHGC, is another factor to consider when choosing energy-efficient windows. The SHGC measures how well a window blocks heat caused by sunlight. This metric is especially relevant in warmer climates or for windows that receive a lot of direct sunlight, as it can significantly impact your home's cooling needs and energy costs. The SHGC is a number between 0 and 1. A lower SHGC means less solar heat is transmitted through the window, thus reducing the cooling requirements in the summer.

However, just like the U-factor, the ideal SHGC depends on your local climate and the orientation of your windows. If you live in a cooler region like Seattle or Boston, a higher SHGC could be beneficial for south-facing windows as it would allow more solar heat to enter, reducing heating requirements in the winter. Conversely, in hotter climates such as Phoenix or Las Vegas, a lower SHGC would be ideal to minimize heat gain and keep the interior cool.

The National Fenestration Rating Council (NFRC) provides an energy performance label for windows and doors, which includes the U rating, SHGC, and other essential information. When comparing products, look for the NFRC label to help determine which window or door will provide the best performance for your home.

As you can see, climate zones are invaluable in selecting the right energy-efficient windows and doors for your home. Different regions have varying temperature ranges and solar exposure, meaning the ideal windows differ in different locales. The ENERGY STAR program provides guidelines for selecting windows and doors based on climate zones, ensuring you choose the most suitable products for your region.

For example, Miami is located in the South-Central climate zone, where windows with a low SHGC are essential to minimize heat gain from the sun. On the other hand, Chicago is in the Northern climate zone and requires windows with a low U rating to maximize insulation and keep homes warm during the colder months. New York City falls within the North-Central climate zone, which prioritizes low U ratings for insulation but requires a slightly higher SHGC to take advantage of some solar heat during the winter.

With its mild coastal climate, San Francisco is part of the North-Central climate zone. This region benefits from windows with a low U rating for insulation and a moderate SHGC to harness some solar heat. Phoenix, located in the hot and sunny South-Central climate zone, requires windows with a low SHGC to minimize heat gain and reduce the need for air conditioning. In the coastal Southern climate zone, Los Angeles should prioritize windows with a low U rating and a moderate SHGC to balance insulation and solar heat gain.

In addition to U rating and SHGC, the NFRC label also includes visible transmittance (VT), which measures the amount of visible light that passes through a window. A higher VT indicates that more daylight enters your home, which can be desirable for homeowners looking to maximize natural light.

Low-E, short for low emissivity, is a term you'll often encounter when exploring energy-efficient windows. Essentially, it refers to a microscopic, thin coating applied to the glass that reduces the amount of heat that passes through the window without significantly reducing the amount of natural light that enters. This coating is made from metal or metallic oxide and is invisible to the naked eye. It won't alter your window's appearance but will significantly affect your home's energy efficiency.

The magic of Low-E coatings lies in their ability to reflect heat back to its source. During the winter, the coating reflects the heat inside the house, keeping your home warmer. Conversely, in the summer, it reflects the outdoor heat outside, helping to keep your home cooler. This two-fold benefit makes Low-E coatings an excellent investment for cold and warm climates. Moreover, these coatings can also help protect your furnishings by reducing the amount of UV light that enters your home, which can cause fabrics, carpets, and other materials to fade over time.

Another factor on the label is the air leakage (AL) rating, which measures the amount of air that passes through a window or door. A lower AL rating means the product is better at preventing drafts and air infiltration.

As you can see, your ideal windows in Austin will be different from Aunt Matilda's in Des Moines.

Let me say a word about the budget. Typically, "better" windows will be more expensive. It may not be worth spending a fortune on top-of-the-line windows if you live in a mild area like San Diego. But if you're in Detroit, your fancy windows (plus possible government subsidies) will likely more than pay for themselves!

In summary, when choosing energy-efficient windows and doors, pay close attention to the labels and consider your home's specific climate zone. Here's a quick recap of the key factors to look for:

1. U rating: Measures insulation properties; a lower U rating indicates better insulation and energy efficiency. This rating is especially important in colder climates.
2. SHGC: The amount of solar heat gained through a window or door; a lower SHGC is beneficial in warmer climates to minimize heat gain and maintain a cooler home.
3. VT: Gauges the amount of visible light that passes through a window or door; a higher VT means more natural light enters your home. Most of us want more natural light (unless you work overnight).
4. Low-E: A thin coating on the glass that helps repel heat in the summer and trap warmth in the winter
5. AL: Assesses the amount of air that passes through a window or door; a lower AL rating contributes to a more energy-efficient and draft-free home.

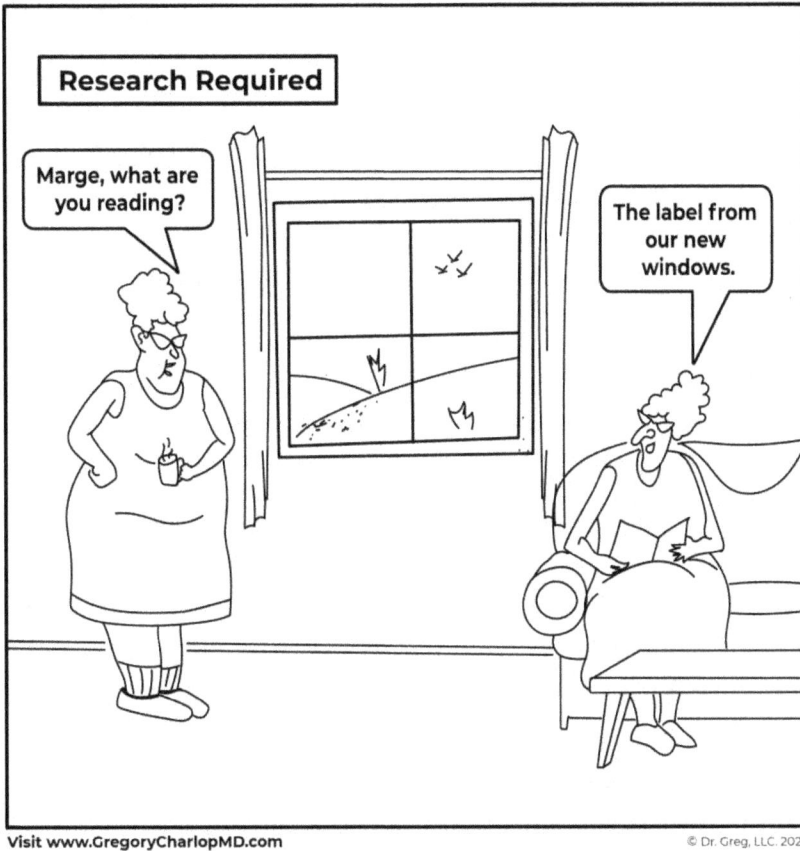

Different Types of Energy-Efficient Windows

Windows come in various styles and designs, each offering particular advantages for energy efficiency, aesthetics, and functionality. Let's take a look at the options.

1. Double-hung windows: These are a classic choice for many homes, featuring two sashes that slide vertically, allowing for excellent ventilation. Double-hung windows with low-emissivity (low-E) glass coatings can provide impressive energy efficiency, helping to reduce heat transfer and lower energy costs.

2. Casement windows: These windows are hinged on one side and open outward, providing excellent ventilation and a tight seal when closed. Casement windows often have lower

air leakage rates than sliding windows, making them a solid choice in windy areas.

3. Awning windows: Similar to casement windows, awning windows are hinged at the top and open outward. They offer good ventilation while protecting your home from rain, making them ideal for wet climates. These windows can also have low air leakage rates, contributing to their energy efficiency.

4. Slider windows: Featuring a simple, contemporary design, slider windows glide horizontally along a track. While they generally have higher air leakage rates than hinged windows, you can still find energy-efficient options with features like low-E glass and proper weatherstripping.

5. Fixed windows: As the name suggests, these windows do not open and are often used for decorative purposes or to provide natural light. Fixed windows can be very energy-efficient because they have no moving parts, which means there are no gaps for air to leak through.

6. Skylights: These windows are installed in the roof or ceiling, allowing natural light to enter and providing a unique architectural feature. Skylights can be energy-efficient with low-E coatings, proper sealing, and the right glazing materials.

7. Bay and bow windows: These styles project outward from a home's exterior, creating a cozy nook inside. Bay and bow windows can be energy-efficient if constructed with high-quality materials and low-E coatings. I love these!

When choosing energy-efficient windows, consider the style and materials used for the window frame and the glazing. Vinyl, wood, fiberglass, and aluminum are common window frame materials, each with pros and cons for energy efficiency.

Wood frames are traditional, offer excellent insulation, and can be painted any color, but they require more maintenance and can be susceptible to rot and pests. Vinyl frames, on the other hand, are durable, low-maintenance, and typically more affordable, but their color can fade over time. Aluminum frames are strong, sleek, and require little maintenance, but they're not as energy-efficient and can feel cold or hot to the touch depending on the weather.

Benefits of Energy-Efficient Doors and a Look at Sustainable Options

Doors are surprisingly important in a home's energy efficiency, just like windows. Not only do they act as a barrier between your home's interior and the outside environment, but they can also contribute to your home's overall aesthetic and functionality. Here are some key benefits of energy-efficient doors and a few sustainable options.

1. Improved insulation: Energy-efficient doors provide better insulation, which helps maintain a comfortable indoor temperature. Superior insulation reduces the need for heating and cooling systems to work as hard, leading to lower energy bills.
2. Reduced drafts: Properly installed energy-efficient doors minimize drafts, preventing cold or hot air from entering your home. This results in a more consistent indoor temperature and reduced strain on your HVAC system.
3. Enhanced durability: Energy-efficient doors are typically made from high-quality materials that can withstand harsh weather conditions, ensuring that they last longer than traditional doors.
4. Increased home value: Energy-efficient doors can enhance your home's value and appeal, making it more attractive to potential buyers when it's time to sell. Your front door is your potential buyer's first impression of your home. Make it a good one.

Let's explore some sustainable options:

1. Fiberglass doors: Fiberglass doors mimic the look of wood while offering improved energy efficiency and durability. They are resistant to warping, cracking, and rotting, which makes them an excellent long-lasting option.
2. Steel doors: Steel doors are a popular choice for energy efficiency because they provide excellent insulation and durability. You can customize them to fit various design preferences, and they often come with foam insulation for increased energy performance.
3. Wood doors: Wood doors are less energy-efficient than fiberglass or steel, but you can still find eco-friendly options made from sustainably harvested wood or reclaimed materials. Solid wood doors provide natural insulation and a classic aesthetic but can be pricy.
4. Recycled materials: Doors made from recycled materials such as reclaimed wood, glass, or metal can be a sustainable choice that reduces your environmental impact. Look for doors with high recycled content and low VOC (volatile organic compound) finishes to protect your indoor air quality.

Federal Tax Credits and Programs to Buy Energy-Efficient Windows and Doors

Investing in energy-efficient windows and doors can be cheaper than you think, thanks to various federal tax credits and programs available to homeowners. These incentives can help offset the initial costs of upgrading your windows and doors, making switching to energy-efficient products a no-brainer. Here are some key federal tax credits and programs to consider when purchasing energy-efficient windows and doors (note: check with your tax professional, as these programs are all subject to change):

Residential Energy Efficiency Tax Credit: Although the federal tax credit mentioned previously expired in 2021, it's essential to keep an eye on any new federal tax credits that may be introduced. These credits often allow homeowners to claim a percentage of the cost of qualifying energy-efficient windows, doors, and skylights, potentially saving you hundreds of dollars. Review the eligibility requirements and consult a tax professional to determine if your specific upgrades qualify for this credit. You can find more information on the IRS website *https://www.irs.gov/instructions/i5695*

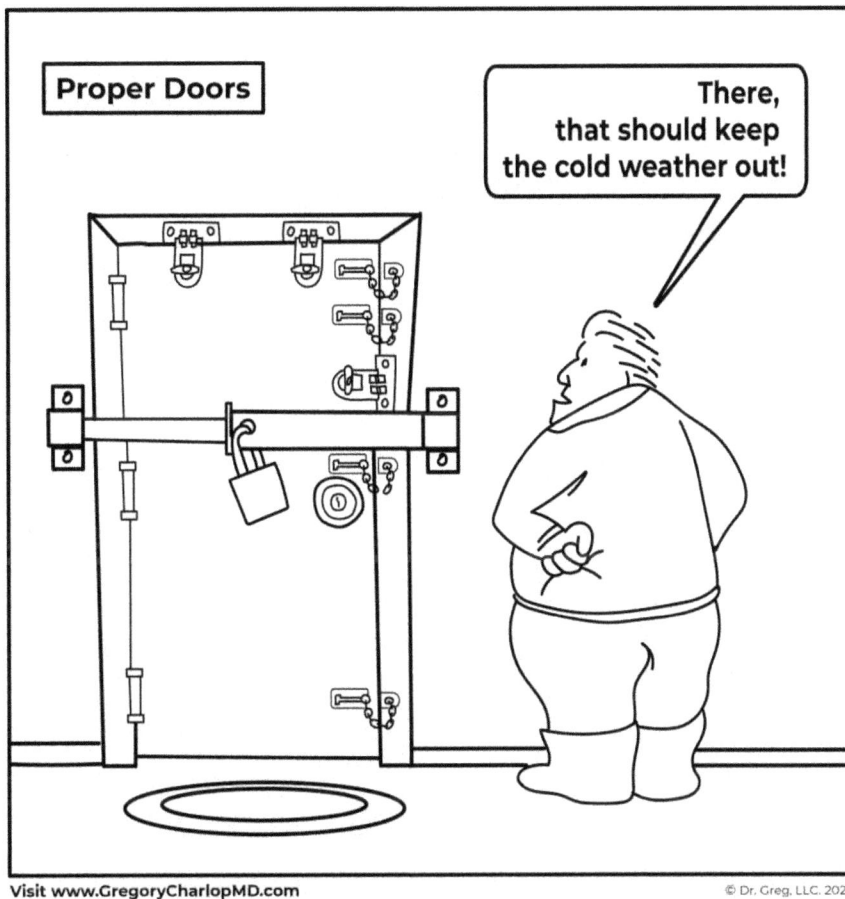

Visit www.GregoryCharlopMD.com © Dr. Greg, LLC. 2023

Energy Star Rebates: Some utility companies and local governments offer rebates and incentives for purchasing Energy Star-certified windows, doors, and other energy-efficient products. These rebates can help offset the costs of upgrading your home's windows and doors. To find available rebates and incentives in your area, visit the Energy Star Rebate Finder *https://www.energystar.gov/about/federal_tax_credits*

Additional State and Local Incentives: Depending on where you live, state and local incentives may be available for energy-efficient home improvements. These incentives can come as rebates, tax credits, or low-interest loans. The Database of State Incentives for Renewables & Efficiency (DSIRE) *https://www.dsireusa.org/* is an excellent resource for finding incentives in your area. Check with your state energy office or local utility company for more information about available programs.

With tax credits and rebates, you can offset the initial costs of upgrading to energy-efficient windows and doors. In the long run, quality windows and doors will save you money on energy bills and will help keep your vintage home surprisingly comfy.

CHAPTER 8

Home Court Advantage:
Top Draft Picks in Insulation
and Air Sealing

Introduction

The stars are shining bright on a cold, windy January night. You're indoors, snuggled up in jammies with a crunchy bowl of popcorn and a good (green remodeling) book. Your living room is warm and toasty, and your pup is curled up beside you.

What makes your house so deliciously cozy? Your insulation.

Welcome to a world where comfort and sustainability go hand in hand. Proper insulation and air sealing are everything when creating a healthy, energy-efficient home environment. This chapter will explore the different types of insulation, air sealing methods, and the benefits of adopting eco-friendly insulation materials in your green home remodel.

What are R-Values?

If you're shopping for insulation, you'll see "R-value" on every package. But what does it mean? R-value is like a score or rating. It tells us how good a material is at resisting, or slowing down, heat flow. The higher the R-value, the better the material is at this job.

Think of it like this: in winter, heat from your warm house wants to escape to the cold outside, and in the summer, the hot outside air wants to sneak into your cooler home. The insulation's job is to slow down this movement of heat. If it has a higher R-value, it can do this job better and keep your house warm in winter and cool in summer.

But the R-value isn't a one-size-fits-all number. It depends on a few things: the type of insulation material, how thick it is, and how dense (or compact) it is. Different types of insulation materials include spray foam, cellulose, fiberglass batts, or rigid foam boards. Each type has a different R-value per inch. For instance, fiberglass batts have an R-value of about 3 to 4 per inch, while rigid foam boards range from 3.8 to 8 per inch.

Thickness and density also matter. More thickness means a higher R-value because there's more material to slow down the heat. And denser materials usually have higher R-values because they pack more insulation into the same amount of space.

Now, how do you know what R-value you need for your house? Well, it depends on where you live. An R-value of 30 to 49 in your attic might be enough in warmer climates, like Florida or southern California. But if you live in a colder place, like Minnesota or Maine, you'll need a higher R-value, like 49 to 60, to keep your home cozy in winter. Energystar.gov has excellent information about R values in different parts of the US.

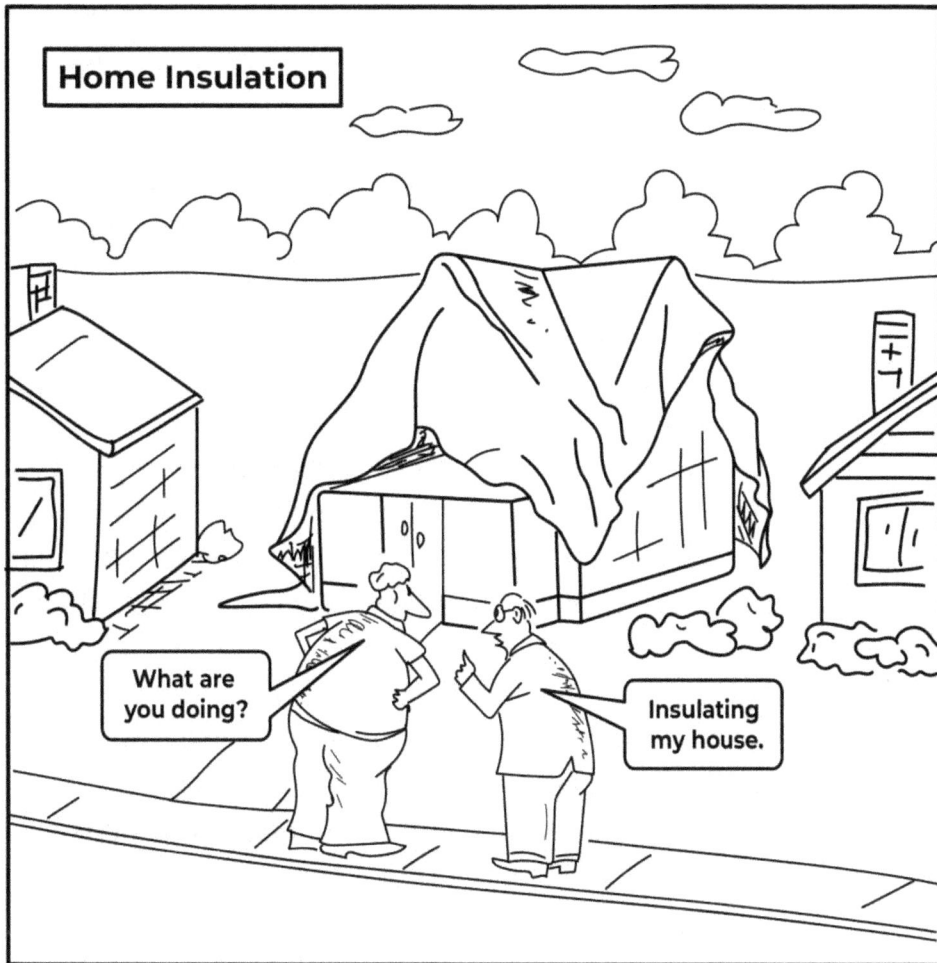

Different Types of Insulation

Various insulation materials are available, each with its benefits and drawbacks. Here, we will discuss the most common types of insulation:

1. Fiberglass: This popular insulation material is made from fine glass fibers delivered in batts, rolls, or loose-fill forms. Fiberglass is inexpensive and easy to install but can irritate the skin and respiratory system if not handled properly.

2. Mineral Wool: Mineral wool insulation is made from rock, slag, or other inorganic materials and comes in batts, rolls,

or loose-fill versions. It is fire-resistant and offers good thermal performance, but it may be more expensive than other types of insulation.

3. Cellulose: Made from recycled paper products, cellulose insulation is an eco-friendly option in loose-fill form. It offers excellent thermal performance and has the added benefit of being fire-resistant when treated with fire-retardant chemicals. However, it can be more susceptible to moisture damage than other materials.

4. Spray Foam: Spray foam insulation is made from polyurethane or other synthetic materials and is applied as a liquid that expands to fill gaps and crevices. It offers excellent thermal performance and air-sealing capabilities but can be more expensive and challenging to install than other types of insulation.

5. Rigid Foam: Rigid foam insulation comes in panels made from polystyrene, polyisocyanurate, or other synthetic materials. It offers high R-values and is often used on exterior walls or basements. However, it can be expensive and less versatile than some other alternatives.

Air Sealing Methods

Proper air sealing is as important as insulation in creating an energy-efficient and comfortable home. Air sealing helps to minimize drafts, prevent moisture problems, and reduce energy consumption by sealing gaps and cracks in the building envelope. There are several air-sealing methods to consider:

1. Caulking: Caulking is a versatile and easy-to-use method for sealing gaps and cracks around windows, doors, and other openings. It is typically applied using a caulking gun and comes in various types, such as silicone, latex, or acrylic.

2. Weatherstripping: Weatherstripping seals gaps around movable components, such as doors and windows.

Weatherstripping materials run the gamut from adhesive-backed foam tape, V-strip, door sweeps, and more.

3. Spray Foam: As mentioned earlier, spray foam insulation is an excellent air-sealing method. It can fill larger gaps and cracks, such as those found around plumbing, electrical outlets, or other penetrations in the building envelope. Full disclosure: this stuff doesn't always look good when trying to sell your home!

4. Gasket and Foam Tape: Gaskets and foam tapes can seal gaps around electrical outlets, switch plates, and other wall penetrations. They are easy to install and provide a flexible barrier accommodating some movement.

5. *House Wrap*: House wrap is a breathable, water-resistant membrane applied to a home's exterior during construction. It helps to create an air barrier while still allowing moisture to escape, preventing condensation and mold issues.

Benefits of Proper Insulation and Air Sealing

The benefits of proper insulation and air sealing are numerous and wide-ranging. They include:

1. *Energy Savings*: Insulation and sealing can slash your home's energy consumption by reducing heat transfer and air infiltration. According to the U.S. Department of Energy, sealing air leaks and adding insulation can save up to 15% on heating and cooling costs.

2. *Comfort*: A well-insulated and air-sealed home maintains consistent indoor temperatures, making living spaces more comfortable throughout the year. Think: cozy winters and cool summers.

3. *Reduced Noise*: Insulation can dampen noise inside and outside your home, creating a quieter environment.

4. *Moisture Control*: Effective air sealing can prevent moisture from entering your home, reducing the risk of mold and mildew.

5. *Improved Indoor Air Quality*: By preventing outdoor pollutants from entering your home, air sealing can improve indoor air quality, which is particularly important for those with allergies or respiratory issues. As a Georgia resident, I sure appreciate it when my house keeps our sticky spring pollen outside!

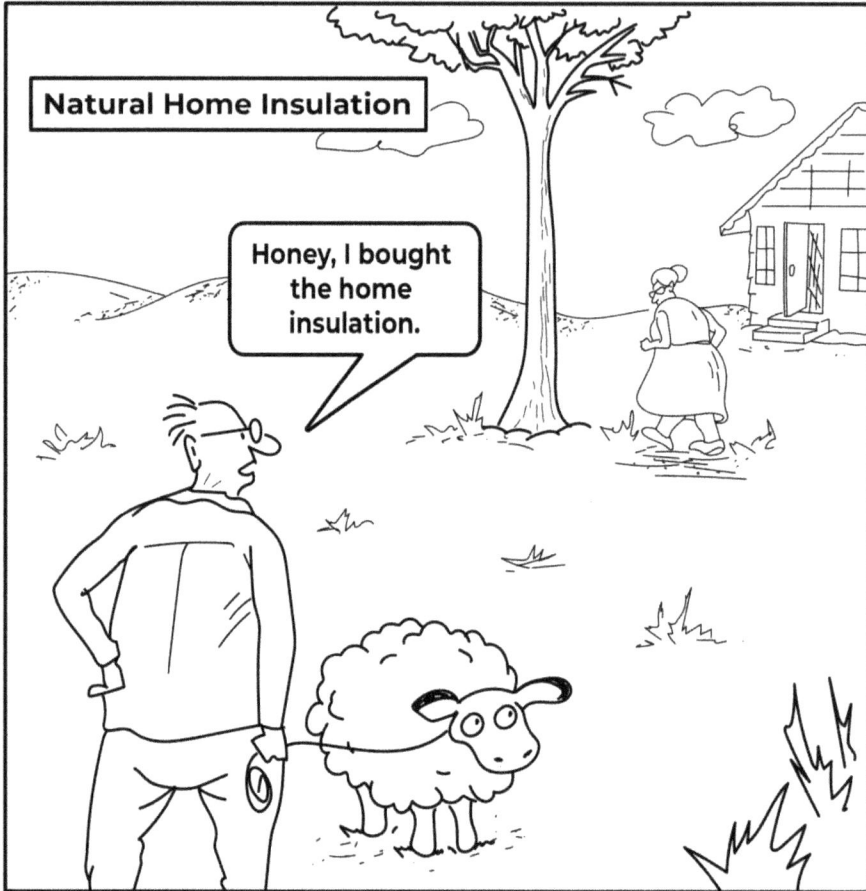

Visit www.GregoryCharlopMD.com   © Dr. Greg, LLC. 2023

Health Concerns Related to Conventional Insulation Materials, Including Mold and Moisture

Let's consider the potential health concerns related to conventional insulation materials. Some of these concerns include the following:

1. *Irritants*: Fiberglass insulation can irritate the skin, eyes, and respiratory system. It's essential to wear appropriate protective gear, such as gloves, goggles, and a mask when handling fiberglass.

2. *Chemical Exposure*: Some insulation materials, such as spray foam, contain chemicals that can off-gas during and after installation. These chemicals may sometimes cause respiratory issues or other health concerns. It's crucial to ensure proper ventilation during installation and to follow the manufacturer's guidelines for safe use.

3. *Mold and Moisture*: Poorly installed insulation or inadequate air sealing can lead to moisture problems, resulting in mold growth. To prevent mold and moisture buildup, it's essential to ensure proper insulation installation and air sealing techniques and maintain adequate ventilation. Have a professional examine any areas of your home that might have mold. You don't want to let this toxin hang around!

Overview of Eco-Friendly Insulation Options

For those looking to create a more sustainable and healthier home, there are several eco-friendly insulation options to consider:

1. *Cellulose Insulation*: As mentioned earlier, cellulose insulation is made from recycled paper products, making it an environmentally friendly option. It also offers excellent thermal performance and fire resistance when treated with fire-retardant chemicals.

2. *Sheep Wool Insulation*: Sheep wool is a natural, renewable, and biodegradable insulation material with excellent thermal performance. It also has the added benefit of being moisture-resistant and the ability to absorb pollutants, improving indoor air quality.

3. *Cotton Insulation*: Cotton insulation is another eco-friendly alternative made from recycled fibers. It offers good thermal performance, is non-irritating, and can be treated with a borate solution for fire and pest resistance.

4. *Hemp Insulation*: Hemp insulation is made from the woody core of the hemp plant, making it a renewable and sustainable option. It provides excellent thermal performance, is naturally mold-resistant, and can be treated with fire-retardant chemicals for added safety. Look for discounts on April 20th!

5. *Cork Insulation*: Derived from the bark of the cork oak tree, cork insulation is a renewable and biodegradable material with good insulating properties. It is also naturally moisture-resistant, reducing the risk of mold growth.

Benefits of Using Sustainable Insulation Materials in Your Green Home Remodel

Incorporating eco-friendly insulation materials in your green home remodel can provide numerous benefits:

1. *Environmental Impact*: Sustainable insulation materials typically take less energy to create and are made from renewable or recycled resources, reducing their overall environmental impact compared to conventional insulation materials.

2. *Healthier Indoor Environment*: Many eco-friendly insulation options are non-toxic, non-irritating, and can even improve indoor air quality by absorbing pollutants or preventing mold growth.

3. *Energy Efficiency*: Sustainable insulation materials often provide comparable or even superior thermal performance compared to conventional options, helping you save on energy costs and reduce your home's carbon footprint.

4. *Durability*: Some eco-friendly insulation materials, such as hemp or cork, have a natural resistance to mold and pests,

contributing to the longevity of your insulation and reducing the need for replacements over time.

In conclusion, insulation and air sealing are game-changers for a comfortable, healthy, and energy-efficient living environment. Choosing the right stuff will keep pollen and pollution out, maintain a cozy indoor temperature, and help you save on utility bills. Now, that's nothing to sneeze at!

CHAPTER 9

The Perfect Chill:
Understanding Heating
and Air Conditioning

Why should we care about heating and cooling systems? Hint: they use a lot of power!

David Bennett, a solitary figure and tech mastermind, had a yearly ritual that contradicted his typically reclusive nature — he hosted an elaborate Thanksgiving dinner. It wasn't just any dinner, though. It was a culinary symphony, an evening of laughter, stories, and shared gratitude that kept his house warm and hearts even warmer. The guest list included his few close friends and extended to his sprawling network of associates, friends-of-friends, and even the occasional lost tourist who wandered into Bennett Lane.

Over the years, David's Thanksgiving extravaganza had earned legendary status. The rumors of his succulent sweet potato casserole, mouth-watering cranberry cobbler, and, most importantly, the inviting comfort of his home had reached far corners of the country. This year was no different, except it was. This year, David had invited a few esteemed individuals from out of town - a renowned tech investor, a celebrated environmental activist, and his rather finicky Aunt Betty. The pressure was on, and the stakes had never been higher.

But as the colorful leaves of autumn started to fall and the sharp chill of winter bit into the air, David was worried. His ancient heating system (HVAC), which had faithfully served his house over the decades, had given up the ghost. He needed a new one, and fast.

A man of the digital age, David plunged into the world of modern HVAC, stumbling upon the realm of energy-efficient systems. They were not just replacements for his old system but an upgrade, offering better performance, lower energy consumption, and a reduced carbon footprint. It felt right. But the question was, could David, a stranger to the nuances of HVAC, pull off this upgrade before his important guests arrived?

In this chapter, we journey with David as he unravels the mysteries of eco-friendly and healthy HVAC systems. We'll explore what they are, how they work, and how they can turn a potential Thanksgiving disaster into a triumph of comfort and sustainability. Join us on this adventure, and you might find the inspiration to embark on your own HVAC upgrade mission.

Heating and cooling systems do more than maintain a comfortable temperature within your home. They are essential for providing a healthy living environment, especially for those with allergies, asthma, or other respiratory issues. However, these systems can also consume a boatload of power, accounting for about 48% of energy use in a typical U.S. home!

In this chapter, we'll discuss various types of heating and cooling systems, their energy efficiency, and how to select the best option for your home based on location. We'll also explore hidden waste within your HVAC system and how to improve indoor air quality through better filtration. Lastly, we'll touch on intelligent thermostats and multiple zones to help you save money and energy.

By the end of this chapter, you'll understand how to make greener choices regarding heating, ventilation, and air conditioning in your home. Let's dive in!

There are various home heating and cooling systems, each with benefits and limitations. Here, we'll explore the most common options and provide a balanced overview.

Furnaces: Furnaces are among the most popular heating systems in the United States. They heat air and distribute it through ducts and vents throughout your home. Various fuels, such as natural gas, propane, oil, or electricity, can power them. The efficiency of a furnace is characterized by its Annual Fuel Utilization Efficiency (AFUE) rating, which measures the percentage of energy converted to heat.

Pros:

- Widely available and easy to install.
- It can be highly efficient, with some models achieving up to 98.5% AFUE.

Cons:

- Fossil fuel-powered furnaces produce greenhouse gas emissions.
- Your unit may require frequent maintenance.

Boilers: Boilers heat water, which is circulated through radiators, baseboard heaters, or floor systems to provide warmth. Like furnaces, they can be fueled by natural gas, propane, oil, or electricity. The efficiency of a boiler is also measured by its AFUE rating.

Pros:

- Boilers can provide consistent, comfortable heat.
- They can be used with radiant floor systems, which are energy-efficient and unobtrusive.

Cons:

- Some boilers may be less efficient than high-efficiency furnaces.
- They can be expensive to install and maintain.

Heat Pumps: Think of heat pumps like a refrigerator for your whole house. They can provide both heating and cooling and are most effective in moderate climates. In the winter, they grab heat from outside - even if it's cold - and bring it inside to warm up your home. In the summer, they do the opposite, taking the hot air from inside your home and pushing it outside, helping to keep your home cool. There are two main types of heat pumps: air-source and ground-source (also known as geothermal).

Pros:

- Highly energy-efficient, especially ground-source heat pumps.
- They can provide both heating and cooling, reducing the need for separate systems.
- Lower greenhouse gas emissions compared to combustion-based systems.

Cons:

- They can be expensive to install, particularly ground-source systems.
- You might need backup heating in colder climates.

Central Air Conditioning: Central air conditioning systems use ducts to distribute cooled air throughout your home. They consist of an outdoor unit (containing a compressor and condenser coil) and an indoor unit (containing an evaporator coil and air handler). The system cools the air by removing heat and humidity, then recirculates it back into the home.

Pros:

- They furnish consistent, whole-house cooling.
- You can combine them with a furnace or heat pump for a complete HVAC system.

Cons:

- They can be less energy-efficient than ductless or window air conditioning units.
- Requires ductwork, which may not be available in older homes or smaller spaces.

Ductless Mini-Split Systems: These devices consist of an outdoor unit connected to one or more indoor units, which provide heating or cooling directly to individual rooms or zones. They are an increasingly popular choice for their energy efficiency and versatility.

Pros:

- They are highly energy-efficient, as they avoid the energy losses associated with ductwork.
- Mini-splits provide heating and cooling, allowing independent temperature control in different rooms or zones.
- Easier to install in homes without existing ductwork.

Cons:

- They can be more expensive upfront than traditional systems.
- Indoor units may be visible and less aesthetically pleasing than ducted systems.

Which heating and cooling systems are the most energy-efficient

Energy efficiency is critical when choosing your home's heating and cooling system. If you score an energy-efficient system, you'll save the planet and some serious coin.

1. Heat Pumps: As mentioned earlier, heat pumps are among the most energy-efficient options for both heating and cooling. They use electricity to move heat rather than generate it through combustion, making them more efficient than traditional furnaces and boilers. Ground-source (geothermal) heat pumps are remarkably efficient, as they take advantage of the stable temperature underground to provide consistent heating and cooling with minimal energy input.

2. Ductless Mini-Split Systems: Ductless mini-split systems are highly efficient due to their ability to bypass the energy losses associated with ductwork. In other words, you're not losing heat by burning natural gas in your basement and transporting that hot air all the way across your house into your daughter's room upstairs. Mini-splits provide targeted heating or cooling to specific rooms or zones, allowing for more precise temperature control and reduced energy waste. Plus, they reduce arguments (and save marriages!) because they let you set a temperature for each room in your home.

3. High-Efficiency Furnaces and Boilers: While furnaces and boilers that rely on combustion may not be as inherently

efficient as heat pumps, high-efficiency models can significantly reduce energy consumption. Look for furnaces and boilers with high AFUE ratings (90% or higher), as these models convert a larger percentage of the fuel they consume into heat.

4. ENERGY STAR Certified Products: When choosing a central air conditioning system, look for products with the ENERGY STAR certification. These systems meet strict energy efficiency guidelines set by the U.S. Environmental Protection Agency and can save you money on energy bills compared to non-certified products. ENERGY STAR-certified heat pumps, furnaces, and boilers offer even greater efficiency than standard models.

5. Proper Sizing and Maintenance: The efficiency of any heating and cooling system depends not only on its inherent design but also on appropriate sizing and maintenance. An improperly sized system will struggle to maintain a comfortable temperature, leading to increased energy consumption and wear on the equipment. Regular maintenance, such as changing air filters and cleaning coils, can also help improve the efficiency and longevity of your system.

In summary, heat pumps, ductless mini-split systems, and high-efficiency furnaces and boilers are among the most energy-efficient options for home heating and cooling. In the next section, we'll explore the hidden waste within your HVAC system and how to address it.

Hidden waste in your ducts and HVAC system

Although your HVAC system may appear to be functioning efficiently, hidden waste can lurk within the ductwork and other components. This waste can compromise the system's performance and increase energy consumption. The following are some common sources of hidden waste in your ducts and HVAC system and how to address them:

1. Leaky Ducts: According to the U.S. Department of Energy, about 20-30% of the air that moves through the duct system is lost due to leaks, holes, and poorly connected ducts. This loss of conditioned air can significantly increase your energy bills and reduce the overall efficiency of your system. To address this issue, have your ducts inspected by a professional and sealed as needed to minimize air leakage.

2. Insufficient Insulation: Poor insulation in your home can cause heat loss in the winter and heat gain in the summer, leading to increased energy consumption for your heating and cooling systems. Ensure that your home's insulation meets the recommended levels for your climate, and pay particular attention to areas like attics and basements, where heat loss and gain can be most significant.

3. Dirty Filters and Coils: Clogged air filters and dirty coils can restrict airflow, causing your HVAC system to work harder and consume more energy. Regularly clean or replace your air filters and have your system's coils inspected and cleaned by a professional. Many home warranty companies offer discounts on HVAC tune-ups.

4. Inefficient or Outdated Equipment: Older HVAC equipment may not be as energy-efficient as modern systems, and their performance can degrade over time. If your system is over 10-15 years old, consider upgrading to a newer, more efficient model, particularly one with an ENERGY STAR certification.

One personal note about the importance of regular maintenance. Some years ago, my heater decided to shut down and pack up shop, just like our friend David at the start of this chapter. The thing was fried. It turns out that the problem was that I didn't change the air filter since I moved in, and the strain on the system was more than its little motor could handle. I had to buy a new machine because of my negligence with the filter!

How to pick the ideal heating and cooling system based on where you live

The ideal heating and cooling system for your home depends on several factors, including location and climate. Different systems perform better in specific environments. Here are some guidelines for choosing the best HVAC based on where you live:

1. Colder Climates: In areas with long, cold winters, a high-efficiency furnace or boiler may be the most suitable option for home heating. These systems can provide consistent, comfortable warmth even during the coldest months. Ground-source heat pumps are another excellent choice for colder climates, as their efficiency remains high even when outdoor temperatures drop.

2. Warmer Climates: For homes in warmer climates with mild winters, an air-source heat pump can be an energy-efficient solution for heating and cooling. These systems are most effective in moderate temperatures and can help reduce your reliance on fossil fuels. Alternatively, consider a ductless mini-split system with heating and cooling capabilities.

3. Hot and Humid Climates: A central A/C or ductless mini-split system can provide efficient and comfortable cooling in regions with hot and humid summers. Solid insulation and sealing will reduce the burden on your cooling system and maintain a comfortable, dryer indoor environment. Look for ENERGY STAR-certified products to ensure the highest efficiency.

4. Mixed Climates: If you live in an area with both hot summers and cold winters, a combination of systems may be the best solution. For example, a high-efficiency furnace or boiler for heating and a central air conditioning system or

ductless mini-split system for cooling can provide year-round enjoyment.

Consult a professional HVAC contractor to determine the most suitable system for your climate and home. In the next section, we'll explore how to use heating and cooling systems to improve indoor air quality and air filtration for viruses.

How to improve indoor air quality and filter out viruses

Your heating and cooling system impacts your Indoor Air Quality (IAQ) by filtering out harmful particles, including viruses, mold, and dust. Let's explore some strategies to enhance your home's air quality using your HVAC system.

Upgrading your HVAC system's air filters is one of the most straightforward and effective ways to improve IAQ. High-quality filters can capture smaller particles, including viruses and allergens. When selecting an air filter, look for those with a higher Minimum Efficiency Reporting Value (MERV) rating. MERV ratings range from 1 to 20, with higher ratings indicating better filtration capabilities. Ensure your system can handle the increased airflow resistance associated with higher MERV-rated filters, which could strain your HVAC system and negatively impact its efficiency. In other words, the tighter (or less porous) the air filter, the harder your HVAC must work to pull air through it. Think of it as sucking down a milkshake through a narrow straw.

High-efficiency particulate air (HEPA) filters are particularly effective at removing airborne particles, but not all HVAC systems are compatible with these filters. If your system can accommodate them, HEPA filters can significantly improve indoor air quality by capturing particles as small as 0.3 microns, including viruses, bacteria, and mold spores. Regular filter maintenance is essential for maintaining good IAQ. Dirty or clogged filters can reduce your system's efficiency and negatively impact air quality. Do you want to breathe air from a nasty old filter? Replace or clean your air filters at the recommended intervals set by the manufacturer.

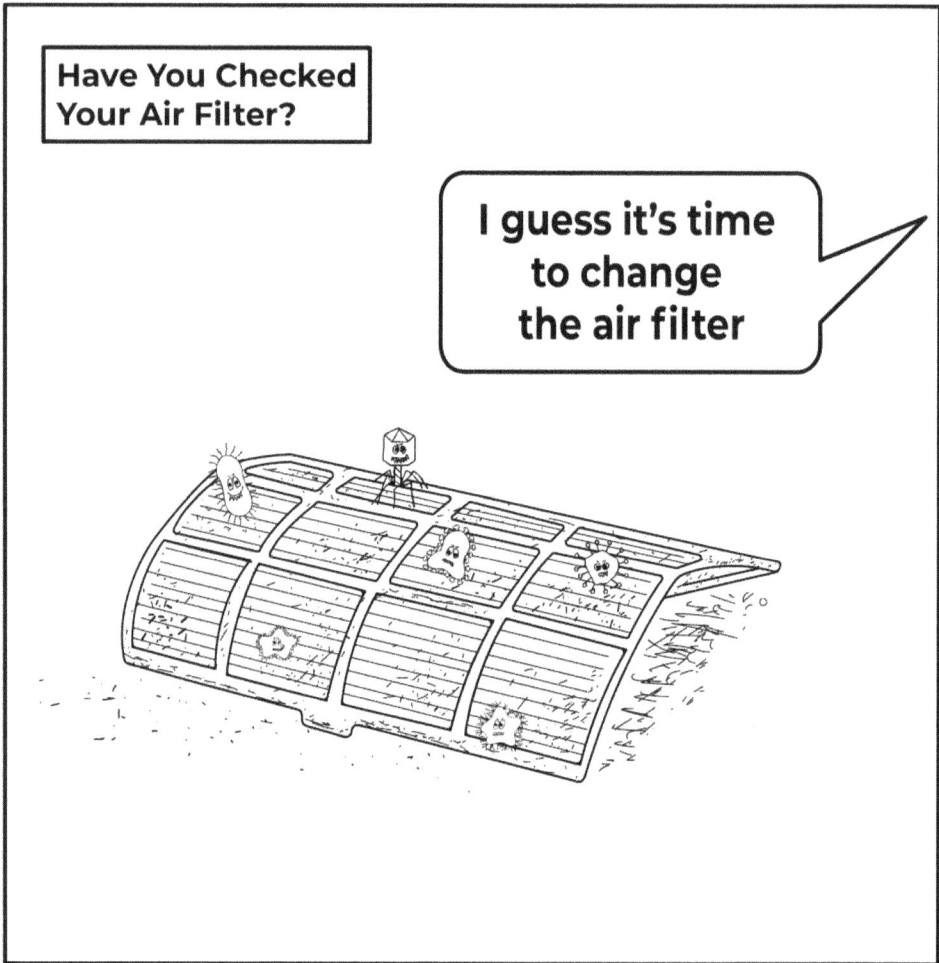

Proper ventilation improves IAQ. Adequate ventilation helps dilute indoor air pollutants and introduces fresh air from the outside. Natural ventilation from open windows and doors can help improve IAQ. However, this is not always so great if the outside weather is terrible or you live near smog. In these cases, mechanical ventilation systems help maintain good indoor air quality while minimizing energy loss.

As a former California resident, I lived near several active wildfires. The smoke from these blazes turned the sun a sickly reddish brown. If you opened your door to get the mail, your home would fill with floating ash. The air was toxic. Thank goodness we had a sound HVAC system! We ran that bad boy continuously to filter our indoor air.

A balanced ventilation system, such as an energy recovery ventilator (ERV) or heat recovery ventilator (HRV), can provide fresh outdoor air and expel stale indoor air while minimizing energy loss. These systems transfer heat between the incoming and outgoing air, helping to maintain a comfortable indoor temperature and reducing the burden on your heating and cooling system. In addition to heat exchange, ERVs transfer moisture, helping maintain optimal indoor humidity levels.

Another technology that can help improve IAQ in your home is ultraviolet germicidal irradiation (UVGI) systems, which use UV-C light to inactivate airborne viruses and other pathogens within your HVAC system. These systems can be installed in the ductwork or air handling units, enhancing the overall air quality in your home. While UVGI systems are not a standalone solution for air purification, they can complement other IAQ measures, such as filtration and ventilation, to create a comprehensive air quality strategy for your home. Be cautious, however, as some of these units can release harmful ozone.

Maintaining appropriate humidity levels is also crucial for improving IAQ and reducing the survival and transmission of viruses. Optimal indoor humidity levels generally range between 30-60%. High humidity can promote mold growth and increase concentrations of dust mites and other allergens, while low humidity can cause respiratory irritation and make it easier for viruses to spread. Your heating and cooling system can help regulate humidity through features like variable-speed fans, which adjust their speed based on the humidity levels in your home. You can also use standalone or integrated humidifiers and dehumidifiers to maintain optimal humidity levels in your home.

Schedule regular maintenance appointments with a professional HVAC technician to inspect, clean, and service your system. These routine check-ups can help identify potential issues before they become costly problems and ensure your system runs at peak efficiency. Additionally, regular cleaning of your air ducts and vents can help minimize the accumulation of dust, allergens, and other contaminants.

You can't rely on an HVAC to solve all your air problems. Since you're thinking about it, it's worth taking some time and auditing your home for contamination problems. Check out your basement and garage to ensure proper storage and disposal of chemicals, cleaning supplies, and other potential pollutants. Clean your carpets, upholstery, and surfaces regularly to help minimize dust and allergens. Bring home indoor plants to naturally purify the air by removing volatile organic compounds (VOCs) and other pollutants. However, be cautious about overwatering plants, as excess moisture can contribute to mold growth and other IAQ problems.

Use your heating and cooling system to improve indoor air quality and remove germs and viruses (like the flu). You can significantly

DR. GREG SAYS

Mold

In the unseen corners of our homes, an unwelcome tenant often finds a quiet refuge. It's mold—a silent intruder that subtly invades our personal spaces, typically drawn to warm and damp niches. It presents itself in various forms—black, white, green, or orange—with a texture from fuzzy to slimy. It's easy to dismiss this subtle intruder, but here's the unsettling truth: it can profoundly impact our lives in ways we might not even recognize.

The news is bad. Exposure to certain molds can impact cognitive abilities in children. That's right. The fuzzy patches in your bathroom could affect your child's attention span, memory, and processing speed. These annoying blobs in your bathroom or basement could harm your child's academic performance.

Bathrooms often provide a haven for mold due to their high moisture levels. To combat this, focus on good ventilation. An open window can be an excellent way to let out the excess moisture, but if windows aren't an option, install a bathroom fan. It's a simple step to keep air circulating and reduce moisture levels, thus depriving mold of its ideal breeding ground.

If you have a leaky faucet, fix it! Standing water is no good.

The key to mold management is quick and thorough removal once spotted. However, the adage "prevention is better than cure" holds water here. Regular checks for plumbing leaks (i.e., in the basement), cleaning damp areas of the home, and considering a dehumidifier can go a long way. If remodeling, explore mold-resistant drywall or paint for high-moisture areas.

Mold and accompanying mycotoxins (poisons produced by the mold) can linger even after you think you've gotten rid of the buggers. According to the Environmental Protection Agency, dead mold can still cause allergic reactions in some people. That means more than cleaning is required. After a significant mold infestation, it's crucial to completely remove contaminated materials, as merely killing the mold doesn't eliminate the potential health risks. The art of handling mold is more complex than it initially appears, and a professional is often required.

Finally, I'm a big fan of home mold test kits. You can grab some from your local hardware store. They let you test the air and suspicious surfaces. You collect your sample and send it to their lab. Before you know it, you'll get a report and advice about how to keep your home safe.

enhance your home's air quality by upgrading your air filters, ensuring proper ventilation, utilizing UVGI systems, maintaining appropriate humidity levels, and scheduling regular HVAC maintenance.

Smart thermostats and multiple zones

Embracing smart thermostats and multiple zoning systems is a game-changing approach to optimizing your home's heating and cooling efficiency. These innovations not only lead to energy savings and help all the picky people at home set choose their favorite room temperature. Let's delve deeper into these technologies' benefits and what they can do.

Smart thermostats are Wi-Fi-enabled devices that automatically adjust your home's temperature based on factors such as occupancy, time of day, and weather conditions. One of their primary advantages is the ability to control them remotely using a smartphone or computer, allowing you to monitor and adjust your home's temperature from anywhere at any time. This remote access provides peace of mind, especially when you're away from home, as you can ensure your HVAC system is working optimally and avoid wasting energy.

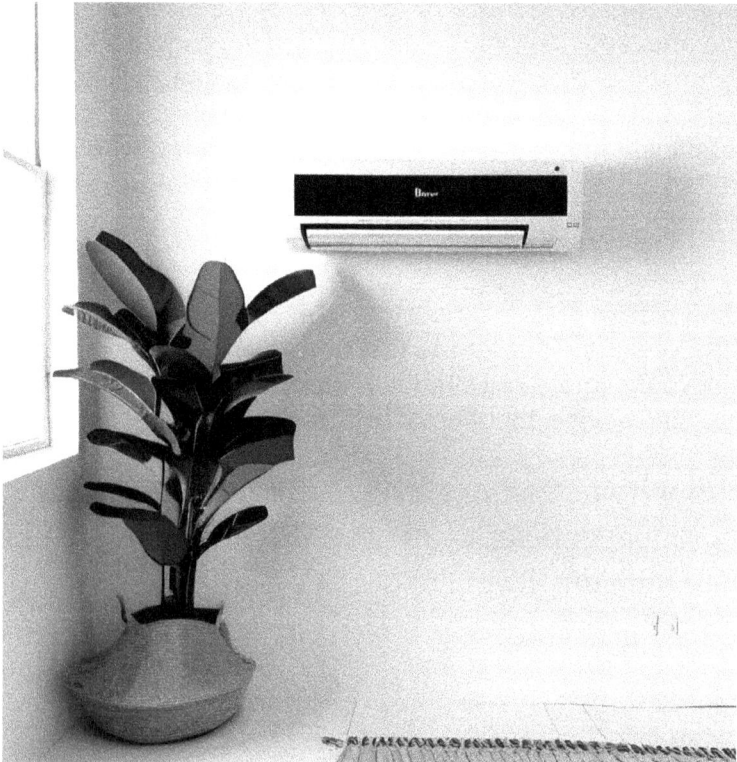

Many smart thermostats come with advanced features, such as learning algorithms, which enable them to adapt to your routine and preferences over time. These algorithms can predict when you'll be home or away and adjust the temperature accordingly. Some models also offer geofencing capabilities, meaning they can detect when you're approaching home and adjust the temperature to your preferred settings. So cool!

Another valuable feature of smart thermostats is their energy-saving tips and reports. These devices can offer personalized recommendations and insights by analyzing your energy consumption patterns, helping you better understand how your heating and cooling habits impact your energy usage. Studies have shown that intelligent thermostats can yield significant energy savings, reducing heating and cooling costs by up to 15%.

In addition to smart thermostats, check out multiple zoning systems. Zoning systems divide your home into separate areas or "zones," each with its thermostat and temperature control. By virtually partitioning your home, you can customize the temperature in different rooms based on usage and preference.

The primary benefit of zoning systems is the ability to heat or cool only the occupied areas of your home, which can result in considerable energy savings. For instance, in the winter, you might set a lower temperature in unoccupied bedrooms while maintaining a comfortable temperature in the living room. Zoning systems can be particularly beneficial in larger homes or homes with multiple levels, where temperature variations can be dramatic.

A zoning system can also help address specific heating and cooling challenges unique to your home. For example, suppose you have a room with large windows that tends to overheat in the summer. In that case, you can create a separate zone for that area and independently adjust the temperature, ensuring optimal comfort without overcooling the rest of your home.

When combining smart thermostats and zoning systems, you create a powerful solution for optimizing your home's heating and cooling efficiency. By enabling precise temperature control and automating energy-saving adjustments, these technologies can help reduce your carbon footprint and save money on utility bills.

As you consider upgrading to smart thermostats and zoning systems, it's essential to consult with a professional HVAC contractor. They can help assess your home's needs and recommend the most suitable products and configurations. Additionally, some utility companies and local governments offer incentives and rebates for installing energy-efficient heating and cooling equipment, which can help offset the upfront costs of these upgrades.

CHAPTER 10

Natural Light, Sleep, and Work From Home Productivity

In the pulsating heart of San Diego lived a determined and relentless businesswoman, Jade. She was a master juggler, adroitly balancing her demanding career, familial responsibilities, and active social life. Late-night work sessions often blended seamlessly into early morning school runs, a routine fueled by endless diet colas. Her elegant urban apartment home reflected her busy life, with bright, energetic lights and a consistently warm temperature that matched the city's perpetual buzz.

However, the relentless pace of life started to show its effects. Jade's energy dwindled, and her formerly-sharp focus blurred. Once a source of pride, her presentations now felt like a struggle. Her work performance suffered, and an anticipated promotion to senior attorney slipped away. The stress began to cast its shadow over her personal life, too. Her relationships drifted.

One day, Jade's world screeched to a halt. To her horror, she dozed off in front of her boss and colleagues during a critical client meeting.

The experience was a wake-up call, as loud and clear as a church bell ringing at dawn. But Jade, a true fixer at heart, wasn't about to let this awkward moment dictate her future. This was her sign, her lightning bolt of inspiration to spark a significant change.

She began noticing how her home environment contributed to her sleep issues. The bright lights in her bedroom, which she had earlier thought were invigorating, were interfering with her sleep. Once comforting, she now understood that her home's heat was disrupting her rest. She finally accepted that her irregular sleep schedule was not worth the price.

Jade decided to reclaim her sleep and, with it, her life. The first step was establishing a consistent sleep schedule—a non-negotiable bedtime and wake-up time. Next, she addressed her bedroom environment. She replaced the bright lights with softer, warmer ones and adjusted her home's temperature to a cooler, more sleep-friendly setting. She invested in blackout curtains for her bedroom windows and chose luxurious, bamboo-based sheets that invited sleep.

The transformation was not immediate, but the positive changes were undeniable. Gradually, Jade found her energy levels climbing. Her focus sharpened, and her work performance improved. She became more patient and understanding with her family. Once a symbol of her relentless schedule, her home became her sanctuary of rest and rejuvenation.

In our hyper-connected, fast-paced world, Jade's story resonates with many. The importance of sleep is often overlooked. However, creating a healthy sleep environment and routine is not just necessary; it's the cornerstone of our overall well-being. And there is always time to start.

Sleep restores our minds and bodies. During sleep, we build muscle mass, fight infections, balance our mood, and regulate our metabolism. A lack of sleep contributes to weight gain, a weakened immune system, and an increased risk of chronic health conditions, such as diabetes, cancer, Alzheimer's, and cardiovascular disease.

Mentally, sleep is crucial for cognitive functions like memory, learning, and decision-making. When we sleep, our brains process and consolidate information from the day, making it easier to recall that information later. A consistent lack of sleep can lead to difficulty concentrating, impaired judgment, and an increased risk of car accidents.

In a way, Jade was lucky that she dozed off in a meeting rather than behind the wheel.

DR. GREG SAYS

Light and sleep

Imagine lying down on your comfortable bed after a long day, ready to get some well-deserved sleep. But instead of drifting off to dreamland, you find yourself tossing and turning, unable to disconnect from the day. You glance at your bedside clock, realizing it's past midnight and you're still wide awake. Sound familiar? Your sleep woes might be related to light exposure.

Light exposure at night profoundly affects our sleep and, consequently, how we feel the next day. You might be thinking, "Light? Really? But I have my eyes closed!" However, it's not just about whether the lights are on or off; it's about the timing, intensity, and color.

As humans, we operate on a 24-hour cycle known as our circadian rhythm, and light is a crucial factor that keeps this internal clock running on time. Circadian rhythms influence our sleep patterns, feeding schedule, and hormone production. As the sun sets, darkness signals to our brains that it's time to sleep. It triggers the release of melatonin, the hormone that helps us sleep.

But here's where it gets tricky. With the advent of modern technology, we've engineered a way to have light 24/7. We can defy nature's schedule and light up the night thanks to electric lighting and electronic devices. But while it's helpful for night owls and late-night work, it poisons our sleep.

Let's talk about electronic devices—your phone, tablet, and laptop. These devices emit a specific kind of light, often called "blue light." You see, not all light is created equal. Blue light has a shorter wavelength and, thus, more energy. During the day, it can boost attention, reaction times, and mood. But at night? Not so much. A Harvard study showed that blue light suppresses melatonin twice as long as other shades and alters circadian rhythms by twice as much.

When you expose yourself to bright screens within the two-hour window before you go to bed, you're essentially confusing your body's internal clock. It's like your body thinks it's still daytime. It's the equivalent of a mini jet lag, complete with the grogginess and lack of focus we experience after a poor night's sleep.

But it's not just screens. Overhead lights, bedside lamps, and even the streetlight peeking through your curtains can have a similar impact. Light in the wrong quantity or color can throw off our sleep.

An interesting study from Dr. Phyllis Zee at Northwestern Medicine exposed test subjects to 100 lux of light (equivalent to the amount of light you'd see on a very dark overcast day). Disturbingly, they found that this small amount of ambient room light was enough to cause greater insulin resistance (a cause of diabetes), faster heart rate, and altered sleep. I worry that these results suggest that over time, even a small amount of bedroom light while we sleep can increase our risk of diabetes and heart disease.

You might be thinking, "Okay, so light's the bad guy. But I can't just sit in the dark!" And you're right. The answer isn't to banish light; it's to manage it smartly.

For instance, limit your use of bright lights in the evening. Opt for dimmer, warmer lights that mimic the sunset's natural glow. Try using dimmer switches or smart bulbs that allow you to adjust the color temperature.

If you can't resist checking your phone or watching one more episode on your tablet, use a blue light filter or the night mode settings. Keep the screen as dim and far from your eyes as possible. It won't entirely solve the problem, but it can help.

The takeaway is this: To boost sleep quality, it's not just about when you go to bed; it's about how you prepare for it. Just as you wouldn't chug a coffee before hitting the hay, you should reconsider spending your bedtime bathed in blue light.

Remember, good sleep doesn't start at bedtime. It begins with how you set the stage for it. With some thoughtful tweaks to how we use light, we can all wake up feeling refreshed, alert, and ready to seize the day. Goodnight, and good luck.

Importance of Sleep for Children and Pregnant Women

Sleep plays a pivotal role in the health and well-being of children and pregnant women. Sleep is essential for children's growth, development, and overall health. It affects their cognitive functioning, emotional regulation, and physical fitness.

Kids who do not get enough sleep may experience difficulty focusing, learning, and retaining information, harming their performance in school. Moreover, sleep-deprived children often exhibit mood swings, irritability, and behavioral issues. Inadequate sleep can also contribute to obesity and other health issues in children, making it even more critical to establish healthy sleep habits early in life.

For pregnant women, getting enough sleep is vital. Pregnant women may experience various sleep disturbances, such as frequent bathroom breaks, physical discomfort, and hormonal changes, making it challenging to get a good night's sleep. Adequate rest during pregnancy supports the baby's healthy development and can help prevent complications like gestational diabetes, preterm birth, and low birth weight.

Implementing healthy sleep habits and creating a comfortable sleep environment can help pregnant women get the rest they need. Tips for improving sleep during pregnancy include sleeping on the left side to improve blood flow, using pillows for support, and establishing a consistent bedtime routine. In addition, it is crucial to address any sleep disorders, such as sleep apnea or restless legs syndrome, which may worsen during pregnancy and impact both the mother's and baby's health.

It's worth having a candid discussion with your obstetrician about optimizing sleep. They likely have some valuable information for you (but might need to be asked!).

DR. GREG SAYS

Teens and sleep

You're the parent of a teenager. You've weathered the trials of infancy, toddlerhood, and all those grade school PTA meetings, but now you're faced with mood swings, rebellious attitudes, and a teen who seems perpetually grumpy. Your household feels like it's turned into a scene from a reality show. Ugh!

But have you considered that your teen's misbehavior might not be just about hormones or a natural adolescent rebellion against authority? What if the root cause is as simple as sleep deprivation?

As countless parents can attest, when teenagers don't get enough sleep, their behavior can take a nosedive. That's not just an anecdotal observation; research supports it too. It might seem like a stretch to attribute the drama of the teenage years to something as mundane as sleep, but the correlation is striking. The adolescent brain is still developing, and sleep is a crucial component. Skimping on sleep can lead to issues with concentration, memory, and behavior. Think about it. Haven't we all felt a bit more irritable, a bit less patient, when we're exhausted?

The consequences of sleep deprivation in teens go far beyond crankiness or an aversion to early morning alarms. The health implications are dire. Adolescents' chronic lack of sleep has been linked to increased susceptibility to acne, weight gain, and weakened immune systems. More seriously, it can lead to heightened risks of anxiety, depression, diabetes, and even self-harm.

So how much sleep should teens be getting? According to the Sleep Foundation and the CDC, teenagers consistently need between 8 to 10 hours of sleep per night. That's not an aspirational goal or a luxury. It's a health necessity, just like nutritious food or regular exercise. As for the best time for them to sleep, this can be tricky due to shifts in their circadian rhythm during adolescence. Biologically, teenagers are more inclined to stay up late and sleep in. While school schedules often don't accommodate this, ensuring your teen is still meeting their sleep needs is essential. (Parents, please encourage your middle and high schools to start later!)

Okay, you might say, *I get it. Sleep is important. But how can I, as a parent, promote better sleep habits in my teenager?* The answer might lie in your very own home. Consider the environment in which your teenager sleeps. Is it conducive to restful, uninterrupted sleep? Is their bedroom quiet, cool (around 68 degrees), and dark?

A dark bedroom is critical for promoting good sleep because it aids the production of melatonin, the hormone that signals our bodies to sleep. When it's light, our brains get the message that it's time to be awake and alert. Darkness, on the other hand, encourages our bodies to wind down and prepare for sleep. Installing blackout curtains in your teenager's bedroom is a simple and effective strategy. Try to get blackout

shades with tracks on the side. These shades block out most, if not all, outside light, even the glow of streetlights or the early morning sun. And this isn't just about nighttime sleep. If your teen's schedule means they're catching up on sleep in the mornings or even napping during the day, a dark room is equally beneficial.

So, the next time you find yourself in a standoff with your grumpy teenager, remember they might not just be acting out. They could be calling out for help—a good night's rest.

P.S. If they don't want more sleep, tell them about the acne!

Sustainable and Healthy Bedroom Design Elements and Eco-friendly Bedding Materials

Creating a sleep sanctuary that promotes restful sleep and supports overall health and well-being goes beyond just getting a comfortable mattress and blackout curtains. Incorporating sustainable and healthy design elements into your bedroom can significantly improve sleep quality and reduce environmental impact.

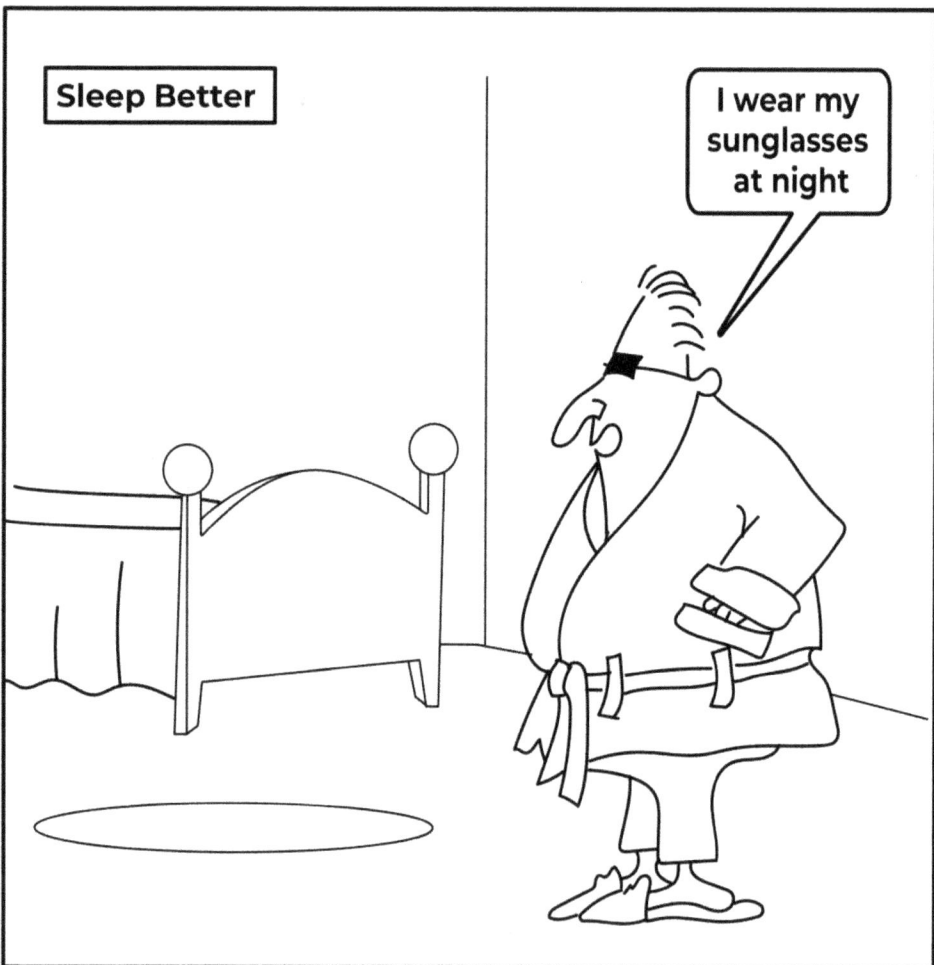

One of the critical elements of a sustainable bedroom is choosing eco-friendly bedding materials. Look for sheets made from renewable or recyclable resources and produced using environmentally responsible processes. Examples of eco-friendly bedding materials include organic cotton, linen, bamboo, and Tencel, which are sustainable but also soft and breathable, promoting a comfortable sleep environment.

In addition to selecting eco-friendly bedding, consider incorporating other sustainable design elements into your bedroom. Opt for energy-efficient lighting and use natural light whenever possible to conserve energy and create a calming atmosphere. Use low-VOC (volatile organic compound) paint on your walls to reduce indoor air pollution and potential respiratory issues.

One more note about bedroom lighting. You don't want a lot of light, particularly bright blue, when you're getting ready for bed. You need something to see at night without disturbing your sleep. I'm a big fan of small table lamps at the bedside. Choose a dim, yellow (or red) bulb that gives you just enough light to complete your bedtime tasks without altering your delicate circadian rhythms.

When selecting furniture, choose pieces made from sustainable materials like reclaimed wood or recycled metal and support manufacturers that practice responsible sourcing and production methods. Adding live plants to your bedroom can also improve air quality and create a more relaxing, natural environment conducive to sleep.

Importance of Natural Light for Physical Health, Mental Health, and Productivity

Natural light is crucial for our overall well-being, playing a vital role in our physical health, mental health, and productivity. Properly timed exposure to natural sunlight (bright when you wake up, dim when you go to bed) will supercharge your work and sleep.

A key benefit of natural light is its influence on our circadian rhythm, the internal clock that regulates our sleep-wake cycle. Our circadian rhythm relies on exposure to natural light during the day to maintain regularity. The presence of natural light in the morning helps signal our bodies to wake up and stay alert, while the gradual decrease in light towards the evening prepares us for sleep. Disruptions in natural light exposure can lead to sleep disorders, mood imbalances, and will turn you into a cranky monster.

In addition to regulating our sleep patterns, natural light profoundly impacts our mental health. A study published in the *Journal of Affective Disorders* found that increased exposure to natural light was associated with reduced symptoms of depression and anxiety. Furthermore, natural light can help alleviate seasonal affective disorder (SAD), a type of depression that occurs during specific times of the year, particularly in winter, when daylight hours are shorter.

Natural light also plays a significant role in our physical health. Exposure to sunlight helps our bodies produce vitamin D, an essential nutrient for maintaining strong bones and a healthy immune system. Studies have also shown that exposure to natural light during the day can help lower blood pressure and reduce the risk of heart disease.

As a quick aside, many folks are low in vitamin D. It's worth asking your doctor to check your levels. If yours is low, you might need a supplement (in addition to sunlight exposure).

In the workplace, natural light can boost productivity and job satisfaction. A *Harvard Business Review* study found that employees with access to natural light in their workspace experienced higher levels of job satisfaction, reduced stress, and increased productivity. I know this is true for me! Furthermore, natural light can help reduce eye strain and prevent the development of computer vision syndrome, a condition caused by prolonged exposure to screens in artificial lighting environments.

Natural light is sustainable. Maximizing natural light in homes and offices can reduce our reliance on artificial lighting, leading to lower energy consumption and a decreased carbon footprint. Strategies to increase natural light in living and working spaces can include the installation of large windows, skylights or light tubes, and using light-reflecting materials and colors in interior design.

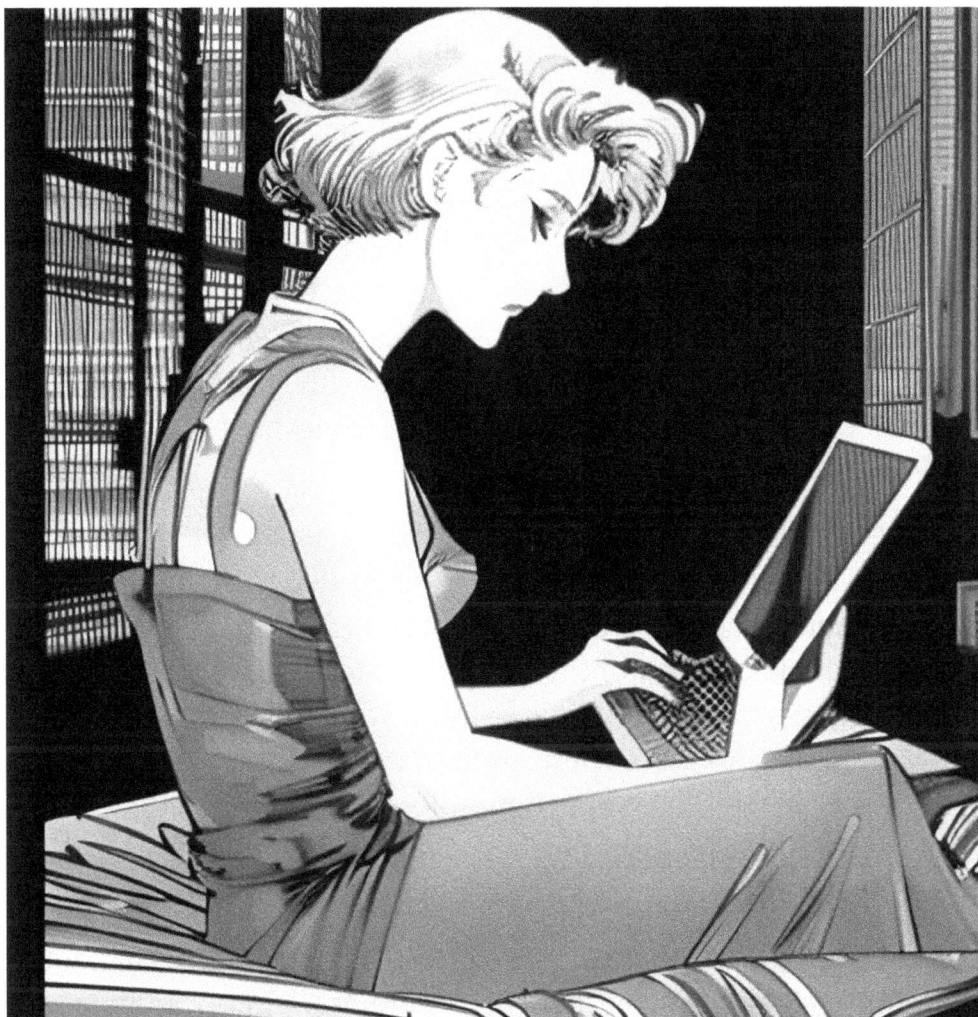

Proper Light in Bedrooms: Bright in the Morning, Dim at Night, Avoid Blue Lights

Optimizing the lighting in your bedroom is essential for promoting healthy sleep patterns and overall well-being. In the morning, bright light is vital for signaling your body to wake up and become alert. Exposure to natural light early in the day can help reset your internal clock and improve your mood and energy levels. To make the most of morning light, consider opening your curtains or blinds as soon as you wake up or investing in an alarm clock that simulates a sunrise by gradually increasing the light in your room.

During the day, it's important to maintain exposure to natural light to support your circadian rhythm and to stay productive with work. Make an effort to spend time outdoors, or arrange your workspace near a window to reap the benefits of natural light. As a doggie dad, I recharge when I take my pup out in the sunshine.

As evening approaches, tone down the light. Dimming the lights or using warm, soft lighting can help signal your body that it's time to wind down and prepare for sleep. Avoid using bright, overhead lights in the evening, as they can interfere with your body's production of melatonin, the hormone responsible for regulating sleep.

Blue light belched out of electronic devices such as smartphones, tablets, and computers is particularly disruptive to your sleep cycle. Research has shown that exposure to blue light in the evening can delay sleep onset and reduce restorative sleep quality. To minimize the impact of blue light on your rest, consider implementing a "digital curfew" at least an hour before bedtime, or use devices with built-in blue light filters or apps that reduce blue light emissions. Keep your phone's screen dim and far from your eyes at night.

Another strategy to improve sleep quality is to invest in blackout curtains or shades for your bedroom windows. These can help block out external light sources, such as streetlights or the early morning sun, which can interfere with your sleep. I got these for my kids' room, and they made a world of difference! They slept in an hour later per day, thanks to the blackout curtains.

In conclusion, creating a bedroom environment that supports healthy sleep patterns involves exposure to bright, natural light in the morning, dimmer and warmer lighting in the evening, and minimizing exposure to blue light from electronic devices. By consciously optimizing your bedroom lighting, you can improve your sleep quality, boost your overall health, and enhance your daily productivity.

DR. GREG SAYS

Light, work, and productivity

Imagine your ideal workspace. Perhaps it has a standing desk or a comfy ergonomic chair. There could be a pot of greenery in the corner (good idea) and a stylish lamp perched just right on your desk. Now let me ask you: How many windows are there in this mental image?

If your ideal office didn't include windows, or a small one tucked away in a corner, it might be time for an update. The reality is that the role of light, especially natural light, in our workspaces and homes is so profound it can affect our productivity, creativity, mood, and even sleep quality.

Remember how your parents might have told you that 'early to bed, early to rise, makes a man healthy, wealthy, and wise'? There's more than a nugget of truth in this age-old wisdom.

When we expose ourselves to natural light in the morning, we kickstart our internal biological clocks or circadian rhythms. This clock regulates numerous bodily functions, including our sleep-wake cycle, metabolism, and immune system. Bright morning light signals our brain to wake up and get going, suppressing the sleep hormone melatonin and boosting alertness.

The impact of morning light on our productivity throughout the day is significant. Dr. Andrew Huberman explained that exposure to bright light early in the day leads to better focus, attention, mood, and even nighttime sleep. We're not talking about a slight upgrade in productivity; it's a game-changer.

A study published in the *International Journal of Environmental Research and Public Health* corroborates these findings. It found that workspaces with windows providing a solid connection to the outdoor environment improved employee mental function and alertness. People in spaces with more natural light reported better sleep quality, physical activity, and increased quality of life than those in offices with less natural light.

As an aside, I left my old job as a hospital-based doctor partly because I worked under fluorescent lights without windows. Winter was dark in the morning, dark driving home at night, and I saw no midday sun. I'd often go whole days without any natural sunlight. Yuck!

Yet another study, this one in the *Journal of Clinical Sleep Medicine*, found that workers in offices with windows had more light exposure during work hours and slept an average of 46 minutes more per night. They reported fewer sleep disturbances and, importantly, better quality of life.

So what's the takeaway here? Embrace the (natural) light.

When planning your workspace or home, prioritize windows that allow plenty of natural morning light. If you work from home, choose a workspace with a window, preferably one that faces the east or south for the morning light. The goal is to get your dose of bright light early in the day to align your circadian rhythms. This is about more than just the view. It's about creating an environment that harnesses the power of light to enhance your productivity, creativity, and overall well-being.

If you have a dog, go out and enjoy a nice morning walk (without sunglasses) before you start working. The early-morning rays will start your day off right and enhance your work-from-home productivity.

And remember, it's not just about adding more light; it's about adding the right kind of light at the right time. Avoid harsh artificial light, especially late in the evening, as it can interfere with sleep patterns. When possible, use light bulbs that mimic natural light's color temperature throughout the day—cooler, bluer light in the morning, and warmer, more yellow light in the evening.

When we talk about designing our spaces, it's easy to focus on the aesthetics: the color of the walls and the furniture style. But it's time to consider something more fundamental, something as simple and complex as light. After all, we're not just decorating our spaces but creating environments that shape our lives. The magic of morning light is there for the taking; all you need to do is let it in.

How to Increase Natural Light Throughout Your Home

Here are some strategies to help you maximize natural light in your living spaces:

1. Use light-colored and reflective surfaces: Light-colored walls, ceilings, and floors can help bounce sunlight throughout your home, making rooms appear brighter and more spacious. Consider using light shades of paint and opting for lighter-colored flooring materials to enhance the natural light in your space. FYI, bamboo flooring is bright, somewhat reflective, and sustainable.

2. Opt for sheer or translucent window treatments: Heavy, dark curtains can block sunlight and make rooms appear darker. Choose sheer or translucent window treatments that allow sunlight to filter through while providing privacy.

3. Install skylights or solar tubes: Skylights and solar tubes can introduce more natural light into your home, especially in areas with limited window space. Skylights are essentially windows installed on the roof, while solar tubes channel sunlight from the roof to interior spaces through reflective tubes. Solar tubes are relatively affordable and easy to install.

4. Use mirrors and reflective decor: Strategically placing mirrors and other reflective surfaces, such as glass or metallic decor, can help bounce light around your home and make rooms feel brighter. Position mirrors on walls opposite windows to maximize the amount of natural light reflected into the space.

5. Opt for open floor plans: Open-concept layouts can help distribute light evenly throughout your home, making spaces feel brighter and more inviting. Consider removing non-load-bearing walls or using glass partitions to separate rooms while allowing light to flow freely.

6. Clean your windows regularly: Dirty windows can obstruct sunlight and make your home feel darker. Regular window cleaning can help ensure you're making the most of the natural light available.

7. Incorporate more glass into your home's design: Glass doors, walls, and room dividers can help transmit light

between spaces, creating a brighter and more open feel. I recommend installing as many exterior screen doors as possible. They're inexpensive to install and are an easy way to brighten up a room without building more windows. Plus, fresh breezes through your screen doors improve indoor air quality. Additionally, consider upgrading to energy-efficient windows with low-emissivity coatings that allow natural light to enter while reflecting heat, keeping your home comfortable and reducing energy costs.

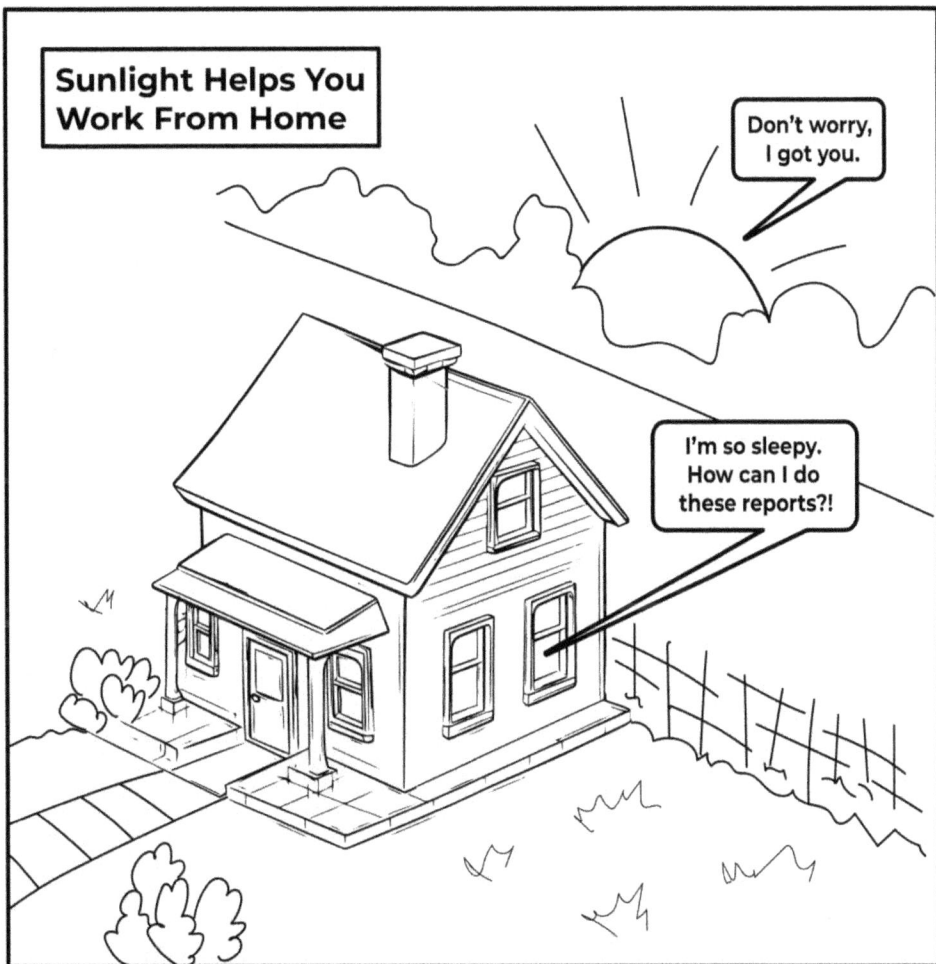

As a sleep and natural light enthusiast, this is one of my favorite chapters. I hope you try some of these techniques and let me know how it goes. Look for me on LinkedIn or my website www.GregoryCharlopMD.com. I'd love to hear your ideas for drawing in more natural light to brighten the day. And if you find this book useful, please take a moment and write an honest 5-star review. I appreciate you!

CHAPTER 11

Glow, Flow, and Grow:
Lighting, Dishes, and Herbs

Last winter, I decided to take my two daughters to the local science museum. As a bit of a Star Trek nerd, I'm always looking for ways to get my girls into the sciences (and away from screens!).

The museum greeted us with a dizzying array of exhibits covering everything from astronomy and geology to biology and physics. We spent the first part of our day marveling at the intricate inner workings of a human cell, checking out every space-related exhibit I could find, and observing the fascinating behavior of foxes in their simulated natural habitats. Since the girls were behaving themselves and not running around treating the museum like an amusement park, I even broke down and grabbed them some sugary cookies. They were organic, I'm told...

After our sugary snack, we stumbled upon an exhibit that caught our eye - energy conservation. At the exhibit's center was a stationary exercise bike connected to various lightbulbs, including incandescent, compact fluorescent (CFL), and LED. The goal was to demonstrate how much energy it takes to power each type of bulb, providing a tangible comparison for visitors.

Excited, the youngest hopped on the bike and began pedaling with enthusiasm. As she pedaled, the incandescent lightbulbs flickered to life, one by one. It wasn't long before she realized how much effort it took to generate enough energy to illuminate the bulbs, even briefly. Her brow furrowed in concentration, and sweat beaded on her forehead as she pedaled. Meanwhile, the eldest started talking trash, itching for her turn on the bike.

After a few minutes, my young trooper stepped off the bike, panting and out of breath, but with a sense of accomplishment. The fresh, new competitor took her place and pedaled just as fiercely, putting her all into powering the lightbulbs. Both girls were astonished by the dramatic difference in energy required to light the incandescent bulbs compared to the more energy-efficient LED and CFL bulbs. The exhibit left a lasting impression, sparking a newfound appreciation for energy conservation and smart lighting choices.

My two tough daughters could barely keep the (incandescent) lights on!

This trip to the museum is a perfect segue into a conversation about clean, green lighting and appliances and how they can impact our daily lives, health, and the environment. Let's delve deeper into the world of LEDs and explore how to make the best choices for our homes.

The Evolution of Lighting

The sun	Fire
1	2
Incandescent light bulb	CFLs
3	4
LED lights	The sun
5	6

LED lighting, but watch the color!

LED (light-emitting diode) lighting offers many benefits that make it an ideal choice for homeowners looking to improve their home's energy efficiency, reduce their environmental impact, and save money on utilities. Let's look at the six key benefits of LED lighting and explore the importance of choosing the right hue for various applications.

1. Energy efficiency: LED bulbs use up to 80% less energy than incandescent bulbs, which translates to lower energy bills and reduced greenhouse gas emissions. This efficiency is

due to LEDs converting a higher percentage of the energy they consume into light, rather than heat, compared to incandescent bulbs. Moreover, LED lights have a more directional light distribution, meaning they focus light where needed instead of emitting it in all directions. This further enhances their energy-saving capabilities, making them an environmentally-friendly choice for home lighting.

2. Long life span: LED bulbs can last up to 25 times longer than incandescent bulbs, with some LED products boasting a life span of 50,000 hours or more. This means that if you use an LED light for 12 hours a day, it could last more than 11 years before needing to be replaced. By reducing the need for frequent replacements, LED lighting reduces waste sent to landfills and helps homeowners save on the cost of replacement bulbs.

3. Durability: LED bulbs are more resistant to breakage, vibration, and temperature fluctuations, making them a reliable lighting option for tough or sensitive situations. Unlike traditional bulbs that contain fragile filaments, LEDs are solid-state devices with no moving parts, making them much sturdier. This durability makes LED lights suitable for outdoor use and in areas where they may be subjected to rough handling or extreme temperature changes, such as garages, workshops, or commercial settings.

4. Instant-on capability: Unlike some energy-saving bulbs, LED lights reach full brightness immediately, requiring no warm-up time. This is particularly useful in areas where quick illumination is essential, such as stairwells, hallways, or security lighting. In addition to their instant-on capability, LED lights maintain their brightness and color quality throughout their lifespan, unlike CFLs and other energy-saving bulbs that may become dimmer or change color as they age.

5. Dimmable options: Many LED bulbs are compatible with dimmer switches, allowing greater control over light levels

and energy consumption. Dimmability enables homeowners to create a customized lighting atmosphere while benefiting from LED lights' energy-saving properties. Not all LED bulbs are dimmable, so be sure to read the label. It's essential to check the compatibility of LED bulbs with existing dimmer switches, as some may require an upgrade to work properly.

6. Improved light quality: LED lighting can provide high-quality, uniform illumination without the flicker or buzz sometimes associated with older energy-saving bulbs. LEDs are available in a wide range of color temperatures and color rendering indexes (CRI), determining how accurately colors appear under the light. High CRI LED bulbs can deliver vibrant, natural hues, making them suitable for applications where accurate color representation is crucial, such as art studios, photography, or retail displays.

Now that we've explored the benefits of LED lighting let's discuss how to choose the right LED color for different rooms or situations.

When selecting LED lighting for your home, it's essential to consider the color temperature and the ambiance you want to create in each space. Color temperature is measured in Kelvins (K) and can range from warm (lower Kelvin values) to cool (higher Kelvin values). Here are five tips to help you choose the best LED color for various rooms or situations:

1. Living rooms and bedrooms: For rooms where relaxation and comfort are essential, opt for warmer color temperatures (between 2700K and 3000K). These warm, yellow-toned lights create a cozy atmosphere perfect for winding down after a long day. They can also help promote better sleep, as warm light is less likely to interfere with your natural circadian rhythms than cooler, blue-toned light.

2. Kitchen and bathroom: In kitchens and bathrooms, where cooking and grooming require good visibility, choose cooler

color temperatures (between 3500K and 4100K). These cool, white lights provide brighter, more vibrant illumination that can help improve visibility and make it easier to distinguish between colors, which is essential when preparing meals or applying makeup.

3. Home office or workspace: For home offices or workspaces, where concentration and focus are crucial, select neutral to cool color temperatures (between 4000K and 5000K). However, if you work in a creative field requiring accurate color representation, consider using high CRI LED bulbs with a warmer color temperature to ensure the best color rendering. I recommend experimenting with different colors to see which works best for you. Your color preference may change with the task or time of day. If so, consider color-changing lights you control via an app. Your goals should be to reduce eye strain, increase alertness, and enhance productivity.

4. Outdoor lighting: For outdoor spaces, prioritize safety and security by using cool color temperatures (between 5000K and 6500K) in entryways, driveways, and security lights. Cool, white light provides better visibility in the dark and can deter potential intruders. However, be mindful of local wildlife and light pollution concerns. In some areas, warmer (yellowish) colors or types of lighting may be required to minimize disturbance to turtles and other sensitive species. Pay close attention to this if you live near the beach. Consult your local homeowner's association or city for more information.

5. Mood lighting and accent lights: Feel free to experiment with a range of color temperatures to create different atmospheres. Play around with the various LED colors, or set up a random pattern to keep your room fresh. Use these flexible lighting options to enhance your home's design, highlight artwork or architectural features, or create a unique ambiance for special occasions.

Wait, are CFLs still a thing?

Compact fluorescent lamps (CFLs) were once hailed as an energy-efficient alternative to incandescent light bulbs. While they offer some benefits, such as using about 75% less energy than incandescent bulbs and lasting up to 10 times longer, they also come with distinct disadvantages.

One significant concern about CFLs is that they contain a small amount of mercury. Mercury is a toxic heavy metal harmful to human health and the environment. While the amount of mercury in a single CFL is small (typically around 4 milligrams), improper disposal of these bulbs can release mercury into rivers and streams. Be sure to follow proper recycling and disposal procedures for CFLs and other bulbs containing mercury. Many local waste management facilities and retailers offer recycling programs to help ensure safe disposal and minimize environmental impact.

CFLs also require a warm-up period to reach full brightness, which can be frustrating for homeowners seeking instant illumination. They may not be suitable for use in areas that need quick, bright light, such as hallways, stairwells, or security lighting.

Additionally, some CFLs may emit an audible buzzing noise or cause flickering, which can distract or irritate folks. You typically won't have to deal with these annoyances with LEDs.

In terms of energy efficiency, LED lighting has surpassed CFLs in recent years. LEDs use even less energy than CFLs, and their long life span further reduces waste and replacement costs. LED lights are also free of toxic mercury, making them a safer, more environmentally-friendly choice for home lighting.

While CFLs may still be a viable option for some applications, the benefits of LED lighting, including energy efficiency, long life span, improved light quality, and reduced environmental impact, make

LEDs a more attractive choice for most homeowners looking to green their homes and protect their health.

Outdoor Lighting

Don't gloss over this stuff. Outdoor lighting is essential to the safety and security of your home. Plus, it has a powerful impact on your evening curb appeal. Consider energy use, minimizing light pollution, and protecting the local environment when choosing your lights. Here are some keys to outdoor lighting:

1. Energy efficiency: Opt for energy-efficient LED lighting for outdoor applications, as these lights use significantly less energy than traditional incandescent or halogen bulbs. Solar-powered lighting is another environmentally-friendly option for outdoor spaces, as it harnesses the sun's power to illuminate without using grid electricity. Look for ENERGY STAR-certified outdoor lighting fixtures to ensure the highest energy efficiency and performance.

2. Light pollution: Excessive or poorly directed outdoor lighting can contribute to light pollution, which harms wildlife, ecosystems, and human health. Light pollution can disrupt the natural behavior of animals, interfere with astronomical research, and even impact human sleep patterns. To minimize light pollution, choose outdoor lighting fixtures that direct light downward and shield it from spilling out in all directions. Proper fixtures reduce light pollution and increase your lighting efficiency by focusing the light where it's needed.

3. Protecting the local environment: Specific colors or types of outdoor lighting may be required in some areas to minimize disturbance to sensitive species, such as nesting sea turtles. For example, amber or red LED lights are often recommended in coastal areas to reduce the impact of artificial light on nesting sea turtles and their hatchlings. When selecting outdoor lighting, research local regulations

and guidelines to ensure your choices align with environmental protection efforts.

4. Security: Security lighting is an essential aspect of outdoor lighting, as it can deter potential intruders and enhance the safety of your property. For security purposes, consider installing motion-activated lights that only turn on when movement is detected. Motion detectors save energy and add an element of surprise for would-be intruders. Be sure to use cool color temperatures (between 5000K and 6500K) in areas like entryways, driveways, and security lights, as these provide better visibility in the dark. Consider adding automated cameras to your outdoor light fixtures for extra security.

The impact of outdoor lighting on animals and the environment

Outdoor lighting, particularly excessive or improperly directed, can significantly affect animals and the environment. Here are some examples of the effects of outdoor lighting on various aspects of the natural world:

1. Wildlife behavior: Artificial lighting can disrupt the natural behavior of many animals, particularly nocturnal species. Birds, for example, may become disoriented by bright lights, leading to collisions with buildings or other structures. Migratory birds can also be affected, as artificial light can interfere with their navigation and lead to exhaustion, starvation, or even death.

2. Insects: Bright outdoor lights can attract insects, which can have a cascading effect on local ecosystems. For example, an increase in insect populations around artificial light sources can lead to a decline in plant pollination or an imbalance in predator-prey relationships. Plus, who wants a bunch of bugs hanging out by your front door?

3. Sea turtles: In coastal areas, artificial lighting can have a particularly devastating impact on sea turtles. Bright lights on the beach can disorient nesting adult turtles and their hatchlings, leading them away from the ocean and toward danger. Many coastal communities have implemented strict lighting regulations to protect sea turtles, including using specific colors, shielding, and downward-facing fixtures to mitigate this issue. Dimmer is better in sensitive ecological zones.

4. Human health and well-being: Besides the effects on wildlife, light pollution from outdoor lighting can also affect human health. Exposure to artificial light at night has been linked to disrupted sleep patterns, reduced melatonin production, and an increased risk of chronic health conditions like obesity, diabetes, and even certain types of cancer.

Minimize the impact of outdoor lighting on animals and the environment by choosing energy-efficient, properly shielded fixtures and adhering to local guidelines and regulations. By being mindful of the effects of our lighting choices, we can create safer, more sustainable outdoor spaces that support the well-being of both humans and wildlife.

Are you washing your dishes all wrong?

Dishwashing is a household chore that most of us do daily, but have you ever wondered if there's a better, more eco-friendly way to get those plates and glasses sparkling clean? Let's roll up our sleeves and explore dishwashing, including popular misconceptions and best practices that can help you save water, energy, and money while ensuring your plates are impeccably clean.

First, let's address the age-old debate: Is handwashing or using a dishwasher more environmentally friendly? The answer might surprise you. Modern dishwashers, particularly those with an ENERGY STAR certification, are designed to be energy and water-efficient. An efficient dishwasher uses about 3.5 gallons of water per load, while handwashing can consume 27 gallons of water or more. Yikes! Using a dishwasher instead of handwashing could save thousands of gallons of water each year, reducing your water bill and your environmental footprint. Plus, your dishwasher will help you free up more time for reading (hint, hint).

Moreover, dishwashers typically heat water to a higher temperature than you can use when handwashing, resulting in more effective cleaning and sanitizing. Hot water helps to break down food particles and grease, ensuring that your dishes come out squeaky clean.

Let's debunk some common misconceptions and dishwashing myths.

Myth 1: Pre-rinsing dishes before loading the dishwasher saves water and improves cleaning performance.

Many folks believe pre-rinsing dishes before loading them into the dishwasher is necessary to ensure proper cleaning. However, this practice can waste a considerable amount of water and is generally unnecessary. Modern dishwashers can handle food residue, and pre-rinsing might make the dishwasher less effective. Dishwasher detergents work best when they have something to cling to, such as food particles. Pre-rinsing your dishes may make it harder for the detergent to do its job. Ironic, I know.

Myth 2: Dishwashers should be run only when completely full.

While it's true that running a full load is more efficient than running a half-empty dishwasher, waiting too long to run your dishwasher can lead to unpleasant odors and dried-on food that's difficult to remove. Instead of waiting for a full load, consider running your dishwasher when it's mostly full but not overloaded.

This will help you strike the right balance between efficiency and cleanliness.

Myth 3: The dishwasher's heat-dry setting is necessary for proper drying.

Using the heat-dry setting on your dishwasher can consume significant energy, and it's often unnecessary for effective drying. Many dishwashers now have an air-dry or energy-saving drying option that relies on circulating air to dry dishes rather than heat. Give them a try. You'll save energy and leave your dishes dry and ready to put away. Interesting note: plastic dishware is much tougher to dry than glass or ceramic. If this bothers you, cut the plastic stuff out!

To further optimize your dishwashing routine, consider these tips:

- Use a high-quality detergent designed for your dishwasher. The proper detergent will improve cleaning performance and reduce the need for rewashing dishes.
- Place dishes and utensils in the dishwasher in an organized manner, ensuring that water can easily reach all surfaces. Avoid overcrowding, which can lead to poor cleaning results. Quick joke. "What's the best way to load a dishwasher? However someone else does it!"
- Periodically clean your dishwasher's filter and check the spray arms for clogs. This can help maintain optimal performance and extend the life of your appliance.

In conclusion, how you wash your dishes can significantly impact the environment, your utility bills, and the cleanliness of your kitchenware. Using an energy-efficient dishwasher, debunking common dishwashing myths, and following best practices can make your dishwashing routine more eco-friendly and effective. Your dishes will thank you, although Aunt Betty may not appreciate your advice!

Growing indoor herbs

Indoor herb gardens are a fantastic way to add a touch of green to your home, infuse your dishes with fresh flavors, and improve indoor air quality. Plus, tending to your little garden can be a relaxing and enjoyable pastime that connects you to nature, even when you're inside.

Benefits of an indoor herb garden:

1. Fresh flavors at your fingertips: Imagine being able to snip a few leaves of basil, mint, or cilantro right from your kitchen windowsill to add a burst of flavor to your meals. With an indoor herb garden, you'll have access to fresh, aromatic herbs all year round, elevating your already delicious cooking to new heights.

2. A touch of nature indoors: Growing herbs indoors can bring a sense of tranquility and beauty to your living space. The vibrant green leaves and delicate blossoms of some herb varieties can brighten up any room, creating a calming and refreshing atmosphere.

3. Improved indoor air quality: Many herbs, such as basil, rosemary, and lavender, have air-purifying properties that can help to remove pollutants and improve indoor air quality. Growing these herbs in your home will create a healthier living environment for your family.

4. A fun and rewarding hobby: Tending to an indoor herb garden can be an enjoyable and educational pastime. You'll learn about different herb varieties, their care requirements, and their uses in the kitchen. Plus, there's something incredibly satisfying about nurturing a tiny seedling into a thriving, fragrant plant that you can use in your favorite recipes.

DR. GREG SAYS

Indoor herb gardens

Like stepping into a rustic Italian restaurant, your kitchen can greet you with the fresh, zesty aroma of basil, the subtle minty freshness of rosemary, and the warm, comforting fragrance of oregano. Adding an indoor herb garden to your home isn't just about bringing greenery indoors; it's a culinary adventure, a health booster, and a journey of sensory delights.

An indoor herb garden is straightforward to start. You'll require containers with good drainage, high-quality potting soil, and a sunny windowsill with at least six hours of sunlight daily. If sunlight is limited, supplemental grow lights can save the day. Maintain a consistent watering schedule—not too dry, not waterlogged—and you've laid the foundation for your green corner.

Let's talk about what to grow. Basil, a classic Italian cuisine staple, is an excellent place to start. Its vibrant flavor and aroma can elevate a simple pasta dish or a Margherita pizza. Besides its culinary use, basil has anti-inflammatory properties and is an excellent source of vitamin K.

Give rosemary a try. With its pine-like aroma, this robust herb works wonders in dishes like roasted vegetables or tofu. Rosemary is not just a flavor enhancer; it's a source of antioxidants and anti-inflammatory compounds that promote overall wellness.

Did you know that certain herbs, like parsley and dill, are natural breath fresheners? They can neutralize strong food odors like garlic or onion—the perfect follow-up for a hearty meal cooked with your freshly plucked basil.

An indoor herb garden can offer more than just culinary herbs. Consider adding herbs like aloe vera, known for its skin-soothing properties, or chamomile, from which you can brew calming teas.

Surprise number two: indoor herb gardening isn't just about taste and health benefits; it's also about mental well-being. According to a study published in the *Journal of Physiological Anthropology*, indoor plants can reduce psychological and physiological stress. Tending to your garden can be a form of meditation, offering benefits akin to mindfulness practices.

From a pediatrician's perspective, this green corner can be a fascinating educational tool for children. It gives your kiddos an understanding of plant life cycles, healthy eating, and patience. From a chef's viewpoint, it's a treasure trove of flavors at your fingertips. And as a gardening enthusiast, it's a mini-greenhouse to experiment with right in your home. An indoor herb garden is a vibrant confluence of health, culinary art, and horticultural joy.

Getting started with your indoor herb garden is relatively easy. Here are some tips to help you on your way:

1. Choose your herbs: Start by selecting a few of your favorite herbs that you use frequently in your cooking. Some popular choices for indoor herb gardens include basil, parsley, cilantro, chives, scallions, mint, and oregano.

2. Pick suitable containers: Ensure you have pots or containers with adequate drainage to prevent root rot. You can choose from various styles and materials, including terra cotta, ceramic, or even repurposed containers like mason jars or tin cans. Have fun with the kids and make some pots out of stuff you have lying around the house.

3. Provide plenty of light: Most herbs require ample sunlight to thrive, so place your herb garden near a sunny windowsill or supplement natural light with a grow light if necessary.

4. Water wisely: Herbs don't like to sit in wet soil, so be sure to water them only when the top inch of the soil feels dry to the touch. Remember that some herbs, like basil and parsley, prefer consistently moist soil, while others, like rosemary and oregano, can tolerate drier conditions.

5. Feed your herbs: To keep your indoor herb garden healthy and productive, use an organic fertilizer or compost tea to provide essential nutrients. Follow the manufacturer's recommendations or consult a local gardening expert for guidance on proper feeding schedules.

With some care and attention, your indoor herb garden will reward you with a bountiful harvest of fresh, aromatic herbs that will elevate your cooking and brighten your home. So embrace your inner green thumb, and enjoy the simple pleasure of growing herbs in your kitchen.

DR. GREG SAYS

Plant-based eating

Every time you sit down at your dinner table, you're not just choosing between steak vs. beans and rice but also casting a vote for the planet's future. That's right; our dining decisions carry a surprising weight in the worlds of land use and climate change! Before we dive in, it's crucial to clarify that my goal here is NOT to discuss the health implications of dietary habits, an arena teeming with conflicting opinions. If you're interested, grab my book, *Why Doctors Skip Breakfast*. Instead, let's focus purely on the environmental footprint of our food choices.

The term 'plant-based diet' may conjure images of strict veganism, but this isn't a binary decision. The idea is to move towards a diet with more plant-based foods and fewer animal-based ones, a change that, according to research, can have a significant environmental impact. In other words, each time you eat hummus instead of a hotdog, you're doing the Earth a solid.

A study from Harvard's T.H. Chan School of Public Health makes a compelling case. It found that the most planet-friendly diets are rich in plant-based foods such as fruits, vegetables, whole grains, and nuts, lower in animal-based foods, and void of unhealthy garbage like sugar-sweetened beverages and processed meals.

How do these dietary choices impact the environment? Let's start with greenhouse gas emissions. The livestock sector, including meat and dairy, is a significant emitter of greenhouse gases (GHG), accounting for a substantial portion of all GHG emissions caused by humans, according to a study published in *Frontiers in Nutrition*. The harm is comparable to direct emissions from the global transport sector.

A comprehensive study published in *The Lancet* offers a ray of hope. The research found that transitioning toward plant-based diets could significantly reduce food's greenhouse gas emissions by 2050 compared to staying the course. Even a modest reduction in the consumption of animal products could result in substantial benefits.

Lack of fresh drinking water is a growing global challenge. Plant-based food production generally requires significantly less water than animal-based alternatives. A more plant-based diet can dramatically reduce food consumption's water footprint, helping us adapt to climate change.

Plant-based diets are superior for land use. Large amounts of land are used for livestock and feed production. If we cut out the middleman (middle-animal?) and eat the plants rather than feed crops to animals first, we'll require less valuable land for food production. Since rainforests are often burned down to graze cattle, shifting towards a plant-based diet will reduce the pressure on our forests and other natural habitats.

Making a difference is easier than you think. You don't need drastic lifestyle changes. It could be as simple as starting with a 'Meatless Monday,' substituting dairy milk with a plant-based alternative, or just going out to enjoy some delicious vegetarian Indian or Mexican cuisine.

CHAPTER 12

Water Conservation Is Easy!

Imagine waking up one day, turning on the faucet, and nothing comes out.

It was an ordinary Wednesday morning for John, a retired Navy Seal now working in the high-stakes corporate world. The sound of a running tap, usually a mundane symphony that marked the start of his day, was replaced by a hollow, echoing silence. He checked other faucets in his urban townhouse, only to meet the same eerie quiet. Something was wrong, terribly wrong.

As a crisis response consultant, he was used to crazy situations in far corners of the globe. But this was different; it struck at home. He called around and discovered that his entire city was affected. An infrastructure failure and dangerously low reservoir levels crippled the city's water supply.

In the following days, John witnessed how the absence of water, so often taken for granted, could bring a bustling metropolis to its knees. A resource so vital, so ubiquitous in its presence, that its absence was not just an inconvenience but a full-blown crisis. Businesses shuttered, schools closed, and hospitals strained under the stress of limited resources.

The county called a state of emergency. The state launched a massive airlift, helicopters thumping overhead, transporting giant bladders filled with water from nearby cities and reservoirs. The military was called in; their mission was now not a battle fought with bullets and bombs but with bottles and buckets of water.

Yet, even with all hands on deck, it was not enough. The sight of dry taps and empty water bottles stirred fear in the hearts of the city's inhabitants. Panic spread as whispers turned into loud desperation: the city was running dry. The mayor issued an evacuation order for the elderly and families with young children.

John, the ever-resourceful crisis consultant, couldn't stand idle. He pulled in favors, called in old contacts from his military days, and organized a convoy to a nearby lake. With a band of volunteers and an armada of trucks, they worked around the clock, pumping water into tanker trucks, driving back to the city, and distributing it to desperate citizens.

Their effort, while Herculean, was a mere stopgap. The problem was bigger, rooted in years of complacency and unregulated water consumption. This realization hit John harder than any physical enemy he'd ever encountered. He knew a fundamental shift was needed, one that didn't just react to a crisis but actively worked to prevent it. Water conservation wasn't just a passing concern but a matter of survival.

As the week stretched on and the city's water supply was eventually restored, the crisis left an indelible mark on John's psyche. The struggle for water, the life-giving resource he'd taken for granted, was now a fight for his children's future. He pledged to use his skills and influence to advocate for conscious water consumption, to ensure that no one had to wake up to an empty faucet again. It wasn't just about making every drop count; it was about ensuring there were drops to count at all.

This story isn't a far-fetched nightmare; it's a potential reality for many regions across the globe struggling with water scarcity. That's why you and I are here today, exploring how we can make a difference through sustainable home renovations that conserve this precious resource.

As the universal solvent, water is indispensable to all living organisms, including humans. It regulates body temperature, transports nutrients, and eliminates waste products. It is vital for a thriving ecosystem, supporting agriculture, industry, and wildlife habitats. With increasing demand and dwindling resources, water conservation is more important now than ever.

The Importance of Saving Water

Water scarcity affects countless people worldwide. According to the World Health Organization (WHO), around 2.2 billion people lack access to safe drinking water, and 3.6 billion people, nearly half the global population, live where water scarcity is experienced for at least one month per year. By 2025, the WHO predicts that two-thirds of the global population could face water-stressed conditions.

Conserving water is not only essential for meeting our basic needs and protecting the environment. Using water efficiently reduces the energy required to pump, heat, and treat water, lowering greenhouse gas emissions and helping combat climate change. Additionally, water conservation helps preserve aquatic habitats and ecosystems, reduces the need for costly infrastructure expansions, and saves money on water bills.

Locations In the USA With the Biggest Drought

The Western United States, in particular, has been grappling with severe and persistent droughts in recent years. According to the USDA, over 90% of the region's land is classified as a drought zone, with more than 50% in extreme or exceptional drought categories. States such as Arizona, California, Nevada, and New Mexico are experiencing the most significant impacts, with dwindling water supplies leading to stricter water use regulations and increased reliance on groundwater.

Thankfully, California's drought improved in 2023 due to heavy rains. Whether this is a temporary reprieve or a durable transition due to climate change remains to be seen. Most experts, however, expect the drought problem to get worse in the future.

Climate change appears to exacerbate drought conditions globally, as rising temperatures lead to increased evaporation and reduced snowpack, affecting water availability. A study published in Phys.org predicts that water scarcity will worsen in croplands globally over the coming century, with the Western United States, Southern Europe, and parts of Australia and Africa among the most affected regions. As drought conditions intensify, it becomes even more crucial for homeowners to take action and implement water-saving measures in their homes.

The Most Effective Water-Saving Appliances and Fixtures

One of the best ways to conserve water at home is by investing in water-efficient appliances and fixtures. The Environmental Protection Agency (EPA) has established the WaterSense program, which labels products that meet strict water efficiency and performance criteria. With WaterSense-labeled products, we can significantly reduce water consumption without sacrificing performance or convenience. (To the builders reading this book: hint hint.)

Some of the most effective water-saving appliances and fixtures include:

1. High-efficiency toilets: Older toilets can use up to 6 gallons (22.7 liters) of water per flush. WaterSense-labeled toilets use only 1.28 gallons (4.8 liters) or less per flush, resulting in up to 60% water savings.

2. Low-flow showerheads: Standard showerheads use 2.5 gallons (9.5 liters) of water per minute, but low-flow showerheads that have earned the WaterSense label use no more than 2.0 gallons (7.6 liters) per minute, providing at least a 20% reduction in water usage.

3. Faucet aerators: These simple devices can be attached to the end of your faucets to reduce the flow rate without sacrificing water pressure. WaterSense-labeled aerators can save over 700 gallons (2,650 liters) of water annually for an average family. Isn't it wild that a simple device can save about two hot tubs full of water?

4. Energy Star-rated washing machines: Energy Star-certified washing machines use about 25% less energy and 33% less water than standard models, saving an average of 3,000 gallons (11,356 liters) per year.

5. Energy Star-rated dishwashers: These dishwashers use advanced technology to clean dishes more efficiently while using less water and energy. They can save an average of 3,870 gallons (14,646 liters) of water over their lifetime.

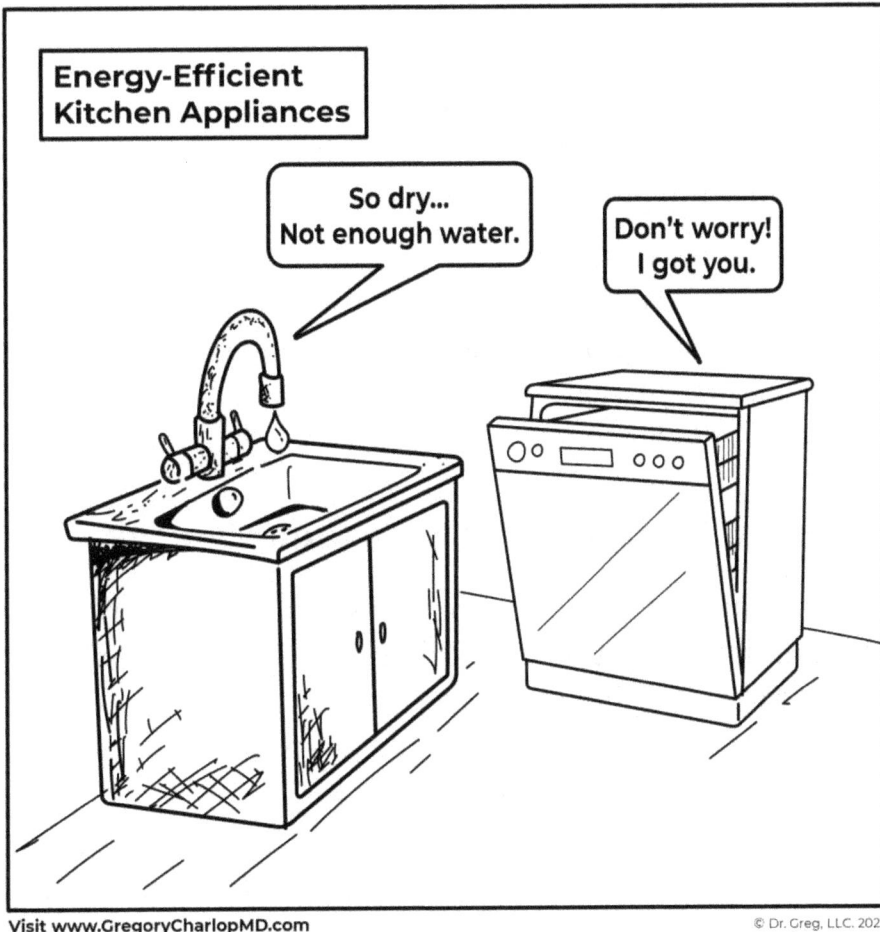

Visit www.GregoryCharlopMD.com

© Dr. Greg, LLC. 2023

What are Rainwater Harvesting and Greywater Recycling Systems?

In addition to upgrading appliances and fixtures, homeowners can implement more advanced water-saving solutions, such as rainwater harvesting and greywater recycling systems.

Rainwater harvesting is the process of collecting and storing rainwater for later use. The collected rainwater is useful for various non-potable purposes, such as watering plants, flushing toilets, and even laundry, depending on the treatment and filtration levels. You can get started with simple methods, such as placing rain barrels beneath downspouts, or more complex systems, including gutters, filters, and storage tanks.

Greywater recycling involves collecting, treating, and reusing gently used water from sinks, showers, and washing machines. By repurposing greywater for irrigation or toilet flushing, homeowners can significantly reduce their reliance on potable water and ease the pressure on municipal water supplies.

Both rainwater harvesting and greywater recycling systems require an initial investment, but they can lead to substantial long-term water and cost savings. In addition to their environmental benefits, these systems can increase a home's resale value and provide a sense of self-sufficiency.

The Easiest Water-Saving Steps You Can Take Today

While installing water-saving appliances and systems may require a significant investment of time and money, there are many simple steps you can take right now to start conserving water in your home. Here are some easy-to-implement tips that can make a big difference:

1. Fix leaks: A small leak can waste thousands of gallons of water yearly. Regularly check your faucets, showerheads, and toilet flappers for leaks, and repair them promptly.
2. Turn off the tap: Don't let the water run while brushing your teeth, shaving, or washing your hands. By turning off the tap, you can save up to 8 gallons (30 liters) of water daily.
3. Be mindful of your water usage: Reduce your shower time, and only run the washing machine when you have a full load.
4. Water wisely: Water your plants in the early morning or late evening to minimize evaporation. Use a drip irrigation system or soaker hoses to apply water directly to the soil, which reduces evaporation and runoff.
5. Choose water-efficient landscaping: Opt for native plants and drought-tolerant species that require less water. Group

plants with similar water needs together and use mulch or pine straw to help retain moisture in the soil.

As we face increasing water scarcity and the potential for worsening droughts, we must take steps to conserve water in our homes. Investing in water fixtures, implementing rainwater harvesting and greywater recycling systems, and adopting simple water-saving habits can significantly reduce water consumption and contribute to a more sustainable future.

Our responsibility to conserve water continues within our household walls. As community members, we can also advocate for and participate in broader water conservation efforts, such as supporting local initiatives, raising awareness, and encouraging businesses to implement water-saving practices.

For instance, you can join or support organizations dedicated to protecting water resources, such as river or watershed associations. Check out river cleanups, restoration projects, and educational outreach programs. Community parks should use drought-tolerant plants and greywater irrigation. Coastal areas must take steps to limit erosion and contaminated water runoff.

Another way to contribute to water conservation is by spreading awareness among your friends, family, and colleagues. Give them a copy of this book! Share the tips and techniques you've learned in this chapter, and encourage them to implement water-saving practices in their homes.

Finally, consider supporting businesses that prioritize water conservation. Many companies are taking significant steps to reduce their water footprint, such as adopting water-efficient technologies, implementing water reuse systems, and investing in water conservation projects. One thing I recently discovered is laundry detergent sheets. They don't use much water to produce and are much less energy-intensive to transport.

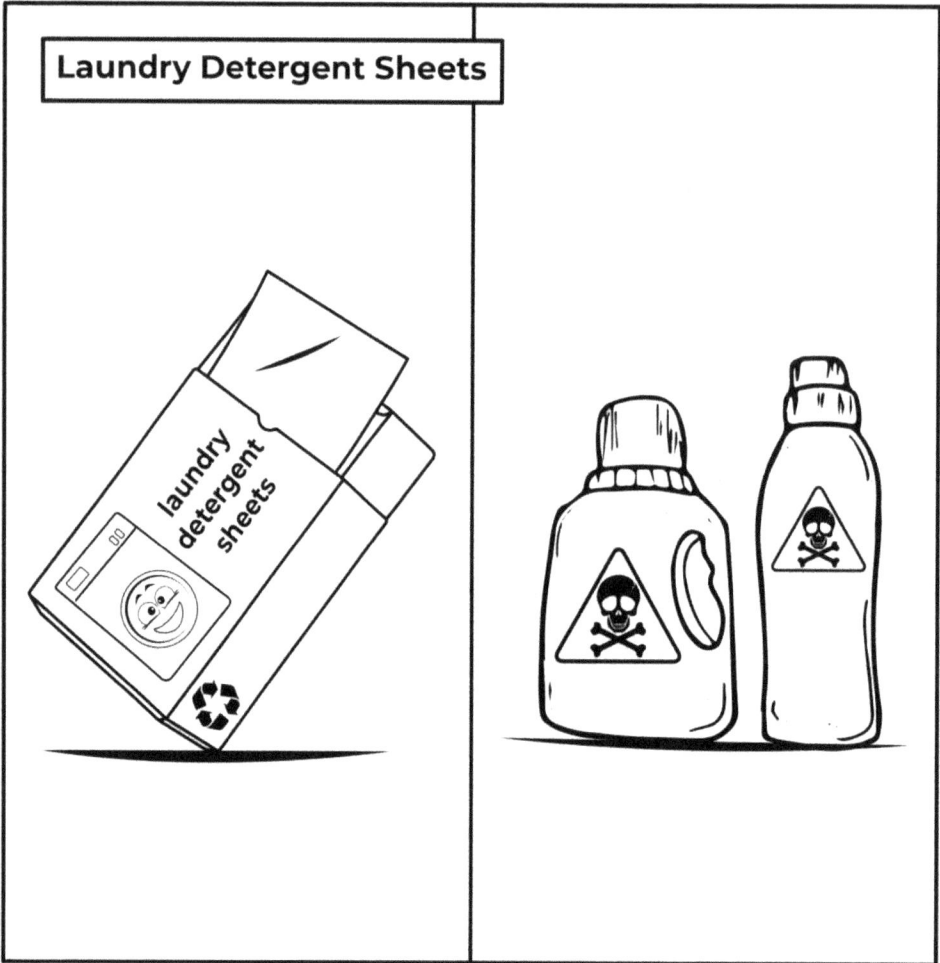

Laundry Detergent Sheets

Water conservation is a shared responsibility that extends beyond our homes and into our communities. Homeowners, builders, business executives, and government officials all play a role in protecting this vital resource for the next generation. Don't take it for granted!

CHAPTER 13

Landscaping for Pets and Planet

Melissa, a dedicated mom of three, struggled to keep her children engaged and entertained during the long summer months. As the summer sun stretched the days longer, her kiddos seemed to grow roots on the couch, their eyes glued to their electronic devices. Melissa was worried, as she knew about the negative impact of excessive screen time on kids' overall mental and physical well-being.

Determined to find a solution to reduce their screen time and get her children more involved in outdoor activities, Melissa tried one thing after another. One evening, she stumbled upon a magazine article discussing the numerous benefits of gardening for children. The author said gardening could teach responsibility, patience, and healthy living. Intrigued by the idea, she transformed a part of their backyard into a family garden, involving each child in selecting the plants they wanted to grow. She even used a phone app to help choose easy-to-grow, non-toxic shrubs.

The family garden quickly became a labor of love, as Melissa and her children spent countless afternoons planting flowers, fruits, and vegetables. The children took immense pride in their work and tended to their plants every morning. They eagerly learned about different plant species and how to care for them. Her kiddos (remarkably) developed an appreciation for insects and their roles in the ecosystem. The garden provided a welcome break from screens and fostered happiness, bonding, and a love for the natural world.

Sipping sweet tea one warm evening, Melissa enjoyed watching her children grow alongside their flourishing garden. She was proud.

As a doctor, I've seen firsthand the benefits plants and nature bring to our mental and emotional well-being. This chapter explores how plants enhance our lives and boost our mental health.

Research proves that exposure to nature positively impacts our mental health, reducing stress, anxiety, and depression. A study by the University of Essex found that participants who walked in nature experienced greater improvements in mood and self-esteem than those who walked in urban environments. And it's not just about taking walks in the park - even viewing nature from your window can improve your emotional well-being. Think about that next time you're working from home!

One of the most fascinating aspects of the human-nature connection is the concept of *biophilia*, which suggests that we have an innate desire to connect with nature and other living beings. This relationship can help improve our cognitive function, creativity, and productivity. Employees with access to natural light and green spaces in their work environments are more productive and satisfied.

Landscaping and outdoor spaces strengthen our connection to nature at home. We can create outdoor sanctuaries that promote relaxation, tranquility, and belonging by incorporating plants and natural elements into our yards and gardens.

Gardening is a therapeutic activity with multiple psychological benefits. Caring for plants and watching them grow foster feelings of accomplishment and pride, while the physical activity involved in gardening can help release endorphins, the "feel-good" chemicals in our brains.

Creating a green space in your yard doesn't just benefit you; it can also improve the lives of your children and pets. Studies have shown that children who spend time in nature experience improved concentration, creativity, and problem-solving skills. Moreover, having a safe, green outdoor space for your pets to explore and play can contribute to their overall health and happiness. I know it does for my pup.

When designing your outdoor space, consider incorporating native plants, which are well-adapted to your region's climate and soil conditions and can attract local pollinators and wildlife. These plants often require less water and maintenance than non-native species, making them a more sustainable choice.

In addition to mental health benefits, a well-planned landscape can reduce your home's energy use and save you money on utility bills. For example, strategically placed trees and shrubs furnish shade and act as a windbreak, helping to keep your home cooler in the summer and warmer in the winter. Furthermore, sustainable landscaping practices can help reduce urban heat island effects. These heat islands are bad news since they cause increased energy use and air pollution in cities.

Landscaping and outdoor spaces are crucial to mental and emotional health. By creating green sanctuaries in our yards, we can improve our well-being, protect the health of our kids and pets, and contribute to a healthier planet. So unleash your inner gardener, and let the plants work their magic on your mind and soul.

DR. GREG SAYS

Dogs and landscaping

For us dog lovers, our four-legged friends aren't just pets—they're part of the family. And just like we'd child-proof a house for a toddler, we want our yards to be safe for our dogs too. But here's the thing, many of the most common plants in our backyards can be harmful, even deadly, to our furry pals.

Let's start with my old nemesis, English ivy. Unfortunately, it's a green staple in many gardens. I've battled these vicious plants for years; they are tough to eliminate! A quick munch on this plant can lead to vomiting, diarrhea, and hyperactivity in dogs.

Azaleas are much prettier than ivy, with their beautiful bright flowers. Ingesting a few leaves, unfortunately, can lead to drooling, loss of appetite, or even weakening of the heart. Bad news!

Lilies, specifically the 'true' lilies, including Tiger, Day, Asiatic, Easter, and Japanese Show lilies, are highly toxic to dogs. They can cause kidney failure in less than two days if left untreated. Yew trees, known for their evergreen appeal, hide a darker side. Their leaves and seeds can lead to tremors, difficulty breathing, and can potentially be fatal. The fifth one on this list is the Oleander, an attractive shrub that can cause severe vomiting, slow heart rate, and possibly death.

Now for the surprising signs of poisoning, aside from the expected vomiting and diarrhea. Did you know a sudden change in your dog's bark or voice could hint at poisoning? Excessive drooling or difficulty swallowing can also be a red flag. An unusually high or low heart rate, dilated pupils, or visible hallucinations are other unexpected signs to look out for.

Creating a dog-safe yard is not as daunting as it may seem, and it begins with being plant-wise. Stick to canine-friendly plants like rosemary, marigold, or mint. Consider these three best practices:

Create clear boundaries. Use raised flower beds, rocks, or fences to create zones where your dog can and can't go.

Know your dog's habits. Some dogs are diggers, and others are chewers. Understand your dog's behavior and adjust your landscaping accordingly.

Regularly check for and remove poisonous mushrooms, a frequent uninvited guest in yards, particularly after the rain.

Sustainable landscaping practices by region

Sustainable landscaping practices are essential to creating a healthy and eco-friendly outdoor space. This section will explore different regional approaches to sustainable landscaping, emphasizing the importance of selecting native plants and employing eco-conscious techniques.

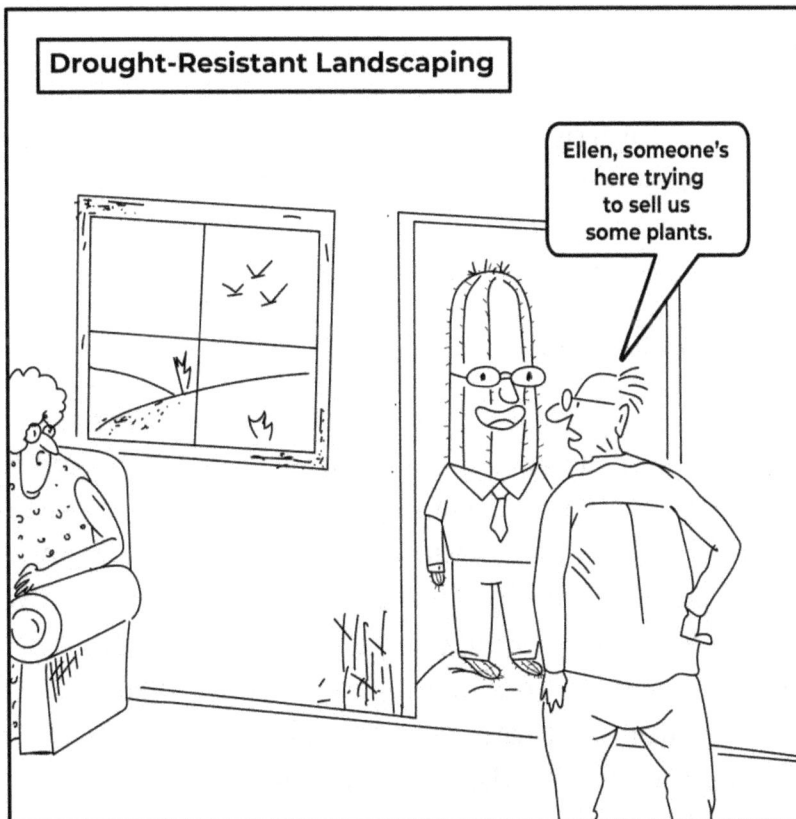

Northeastern United States:

In this region, sustainable gardening practices use native plants that can withstand cold winters and thrive in various soil types. Examples of native plants include the eastern redbud, dogwood, certain fern species, and wildflowers like columbine and asters. To support biodiversity, consider incorporating plants that provide food and shelter for local wildlife, such as berry-producing shrubs and trees with cavities for nesting. Rain gardens, which help manage stormwater runoff and prevent erosion, are useful in the Northeast. These gardens often include water-tolerant plants like Joe Pye weed, swamp milkweed, and various sedges.

Southeastern United States:

The Southeast is known for its warm, humid climate. Gardeners here often choose native plants that can tolerate heat and humidity, such as the southern magnolia, azalea, beautyberry, and bald cypress. To conserve water, consider planting drought-tolerant species like muhly grass and yucca. Try using rain barrels to collect water for irrigation. Also, be mindful of the region's high humidity, which can promote the growth of mold and mildew. Choose plants with good air circulation and disease resistance to minimize the need for chemical treatments.

Midwestern United States:

The Midwest is characterized by its vast prairies and grasslands, so incorporating native grasses like little bluestem, prairie dropseed, and switchgrass is essential. These grasses can provide excellent ground cover, prevent soil erosion, and create a visually appealing landscape. The region is also known for its colorful wildflowers, such as purple coneflower, black-eyed Susan, and butterfly milkweed, which attract pollinators and support local ecosystems. To conserve water and protect water quality, use mulch to retain soil moisture, prevent weeds, and minimize the need for chemical herbicides. Additionally, consider incorporating buffer strips, vegetated areas near bodies of water that help filter runoff and prevent pollutants from entering streams and rivers.

Western United States:

In the arid Western states, sustainable landscaping focuses on water conservation and the use of native, drought-tolerant plants. Popular options include succulents like agave, aloe, desert-adapted trees, and shrubs like palo verde, mesquite, and creosote bush. Xeriscaping, a landscaping technique emphasizing water conservation, is a powerful tool out West. Methods include drip irrigation, grouping plants with similar water needs, and covering the soil with mulch or gravel to reduce evaporation. Additionally, creating wildlife-friendly habitats with native plants can support the region's unique biodiversity, such as hummingbirds, lizards, and desert tortoises.

The birds, butterflies, and bees

Creating a pollinator-friendly garden is vital to sustainable landscaping. Pollinators, such as bees, butterflies, and hummingbirds, play a crucial role in the reproduction of many plants, including the fruits and vegetables we eat. Attracting these creatures to your yard contributes to your garden's health and supports the larger ecosystem. Here are some strategies for creating a pollinator-friendly garden that also attracts birds:

1. Plant diversity: Include a wide variety of flowering plants to attract different pollinators and provide a continuous food source throughout the growing season. Choose plants with different blooming periods, flower shapes, and colors, ensuring something is always in bloom. Native plants like milkweed, coneflowers, and asters are excellent choices that support pollinators and are well-adapted to your region's climate and soil conditions.

2. Layer your landscape: Space permitting, design your garden with multiple layers to create diverse habitats for various

species. Try combining ground covers, herbaceous plants, shrubs, and trees, providing shelter and nesting opportunities for birds and pollinators. For example, ground-nesting bees need bare soil patches, while cavity-nesting birds require trees or shrubs with enough space.

3. Provide food sources: Besides nectar-rich flowers for pollinators, consider planting fruit- and seed-bearing plants to attract birds. Examples include berry-producing shrubs like serviceberry, chokeberry, and elderberry and seed-producing plants like sunflowers, coneflowers, and native grasses. Bird feeders stocked with seeds, suet, or nectar can also provide supplemental food for birds, especially during the winter months.

4. Water sources: Supplying a consistent source of fresh water is crucial for pollinators and birds. A shallow birdbath, pond, or water feature can be a valuable addition to your garden, providing a place for pollinators and birds to drink and bathe. To prevent the spread of diseases and keep the water fresh, clean and refill your water sources regularly.

5. Avoid pesticides: Chemical pesticides can harm pollinators and birds, so opt for organic and non-toxic methods to control pests in your garden. Instead, use natural pest control strategies, such as attracting beneficial insects, like ladybugs and lacewings, or using insecticidal soaps and oils that are less harmful to pollinators. Be cautious with store-bought ladybugs, as they are sometimes harvested cruelly. Encouraging natural predators, such as birds, bats, and frogs, can also help keep pest populations in check.

6. Create nesting and shelter sites: Provide nesting materials and safe spaces for pollinators and birds to raise their young. Many bee species require cavities in wood, while butterflies need specific host plants for their caterpillars to feed on, such as milkweed for monarch butterflies. For birds, consider installing birdhouses designed for native species or

leaving dead trees standing, as they provide natural nesting cavities and attract insect prey.

7. Maintain a wildlife-friendly yard: Minimize chemicals, mow your lawn less frequently, and leave some leaf litter on the ground to create a more hospitable environment for pollinators, birds, and other wildlife. These practices provide essential habitat and food sources for various species while reducing your yard's environmental impact.

You can create a vibrant, pollinator-friendly garden that supports local ecosystems and benefits the health of your plants. Your yard will become a haven for birds, butterflies, and bees.

DR. GREG SAYS

Natural Pesticides

The Smarter Way to Battle Bugs: A Guide to Healthy, Safer, and Eco-Friendly Home Pesticides

Pests can be a real pain in the proverbial behind, whether it's ants marching one by one onto your kitchen countertop or mosquitoes treating you like an all-you-can-eat buffet. Traditional pesticides often seem the easiest solution, but these chemical warriors carry hidden costs. They can harm children and pets, destroy the biodiversity in your backyard, and even threaten your health. Moreover, they're no friends to bees and other pollinators essential for plant life.

The good news is that eco-friendly pest control methods are coming into their own, offering safer and more sustainable options. They may require more effort, but the trade-off is worth it. So, let's explore these beneficial bug battlers.

The Power of Plants

Some plants are natural insect deterrents. Marigolds, for example, produce a compound called alpha-terthienyl (tertiophene) that's toxic to nematodes, small worms that can damage garden plants. Growing these vibrant flowers around the edge of your garden creates a defensive perimeter.

The strong aroma of mint wards off pests. Mint oil sprays can deter ants, fleas, and even rodents. However, if you choose to plant mint, remember it's a fast spreader. Try planting it in a pot sunk into the ground to keep it from taking over.

Biological Control Agents

Biological control agents are another fantastic option. Now, I know what you're thinking: "Dr. Greg, you want me to introduce more bugs to get rid of bugs?" Stick with me. This method involves using the pests' natural enemies to control them. Think of it as turning the food chain to your advantage. For example, ladybugs and spiders are predatory bugs that feast on common garden pests. Similarly, parasitic wasps lay their eggs in pests, eventually leading to the host's demise. Before investing in these critters, be sure to chat with your local landscape expert and only choose bugs native to your area. It's a bug-eat-bug world out there, folks!

Eco-Friendly Pesticides

If you're still keen on using pesticides, let's explore the greener side of the spectrum. Consider biopesticides made from naturally occurring substances or microbial pesticides, which use microorganisms to control pests. For instance, there's a bacterium called Bacillus thuringiensis (Bt for short because, who can pronounce that, right?), which is used against mosquitoes and caterpillars but doesn't harm birds, mammals, or most beneficial insects.

Garlic-Insecticide Spray: Garlic isn't just good for warding off vampires; it's also effective against insects. You can make a natural insecticide using garlic, water, and a dollop of dish soap. Blend two whole bulbs (not just two cloves) with a small amount of water, then strain it and add enough water to make a gallon of garlic water. Add a few drops of eco-friendly dish soap, which helps the mixture stick to the leaves of your plants. This spray can combat aphids, whiteflies, and many beetles. But remember not to apply it on a hot, sunny day to avoid burning your plants.

Hot Pepper Spray: This spray can deter a variety of pests. Blend two cups of hot peppers (the hotter, the better) with a gallon of water and let it steep overnight. Strain the mixture and spray it on your plants. But be careful: always wear gloves when handling hot peppers or the spray made from them, and avoid getting it in your eyes or on your skin.

These homemade sprays are safer around children and pets and are kinder to the environment than many commercial pesticides. As with any pest control product, use them mindfully to avoid harming beneficial insects.

Smart Home Practices

Finally, remember that prevention is better than cure. Simple home practices can go a long way in keeping pests at bay. Seal gaps in doors and windows to keep bugs out. Store your food properly, and don't leave water standing. Pests, like all creatures, need food and water to survive. So, by cutting off their supply, you're making your home a whole lot less appealing.

It's essential to remember that our goal isn't to create a bug-free utopia. Insects are crucial in the ecosystem, from breaking down waste to pollinating plants. We want balance, a way to coexist without having our homes and gardens overrun.

While it might take some trial and error to find the right eco-friendly pest control solution for you, the benefits are worth the effort. You'll create a healthier environment for you and your family, and help preserve our ecosystems. And hey, even if you only manage to convince a few of your ants to picnic elsewhere, that's a step in the right direction.

Non-toxic ways to keep mosquitoes at bay

While you want to welcome pollinators and birds, you won't be so happy if your backyard is infested with bloodsucking bugs. Mosquitoes are a nuisance and can transmit diseases like West Nile and Zika. Instead of using toxic chemicals, consider these eco-friendly and non-toxic methods to control mosquitoes in your yard:

1. Remove standing water: Mosquitoes lay their eggs in standing water, so eliminating these breeding sites is the first step in controlling their population. If you have a pond or water feature, consider adding mosquito-eating fish like goldfish or guppies. Use a pond aerator to keep the water

moving and discourage mosquito breeding. Empty birdbaths, flowerpot saucers, and other containers regularly, and make sure your gutters are clean and debris-free.

2. Natural mosquito-repellent plants: Planting mosquito-repelling plants in your garden can help deter these pests. Examples include citronella, lemon balm, marigolds, and catnip. While these plants alone may not be enough to eliminate mosquitoes, they can help reduce their numbers when combined with other strategies.

3. Encourage natural predators: Many animals, such as birds, bats, frogs, and dragonflies, feed on mosquitoes and can help keep their populations in check. To attract these predators, provide suitable habitats and food sources. For example, install a bat house for bats, create a small pond or water feature for frogs and dragonflies, and plant native vegetation to provide bird shelter and nesting sites.

4. Use fans: Mosquitoes are weak fliers, and a strong breeze can make it difficult for them to land and bite. Position outdoor fans near seating areas to create a mosquito-free zone during outdoor gatherings.

5. Install screens: Ensure windows and doors are equipped with tight-fitting screens to prevent mosquitoes from entering your home. Repair any holes or tears to ensure they effectively keep mosquitoes out.

6. Non-toxic mosquito traps: Several non-toxic mosquito traps are available on the market to help reduce mosquito populations without harming the environment. These traps typically use a combination of heat, light, or carbon dioxide to attract mosquitoes and then trap them in a container or on a sticky surface.

7. Personal protection: When spending time outdoors, especially during the peak mosquito activity times of dawn and dusk, wear long sleeves and pants, apply a non-toxic mosquito repellent, and use mosquito netting over beds or seating areas.

Top five Eco-friendly hardscape materials

When designing your outdoor space, choose environmentally friendly hardscape materials that minimize environmental impact and complement your green landscaping efforts. Here are five eco-friendly hardscape materials to consider for your next project:

1. Permeable paving: Permeable paving materials, like porous concrete, allow water to pass through their surface and infiltrate into the ground below. Permeable paving is an excellent choice for patios, driveways, and walkways, especially in areas with heavy rainfall or poor drainage. These hardscapes reduce stormwater runoff, minimize flooding risk, and replenish groundwater supplies.

2. Recycled materials: Using recycled materials in your hardscape projects reduces waste and conserves natural resources. Consider using materials like recycled brick, reclaimed lumber, or rubber mulch for your next project. These materials can be used for pathways, retaining walls, and other structures, providing an eco-friendly and visually appealing alternative to traditional hardscape materials.

3. Natural stone: Natural stone is a durable, low-maintenance, versatile hardscape material. When sourced from local quarries, natural stone has a smaller carbon footprint than materials requiring significant processing and transportation. When choosing natural stone for your hardscape project, look for locally sourced options like flagstone, limestone, or slate, which have a minimal environmental impact.

4. Composite decking: Made from recycled plastic and wood fibers, composite decking is a sustainable alternative to traditional wood decking. It is durable, low-maintenance, and resistant to rot, insects, and fading. By choosing composite decking, you're reducing the demand for virgin wood and repurposing plastic waste that would otherwise end up in landfills.

5. Gravel and crushed stone: Gravel and crushed stone are affordable, low-impact hardscape materials that you can use for pathways, patios, and driveways. They are permeable, allowing water to infiltrate the ground and reduce stormwater runoff, and when locally sourced, minimize the environmental impact associated with transportation.

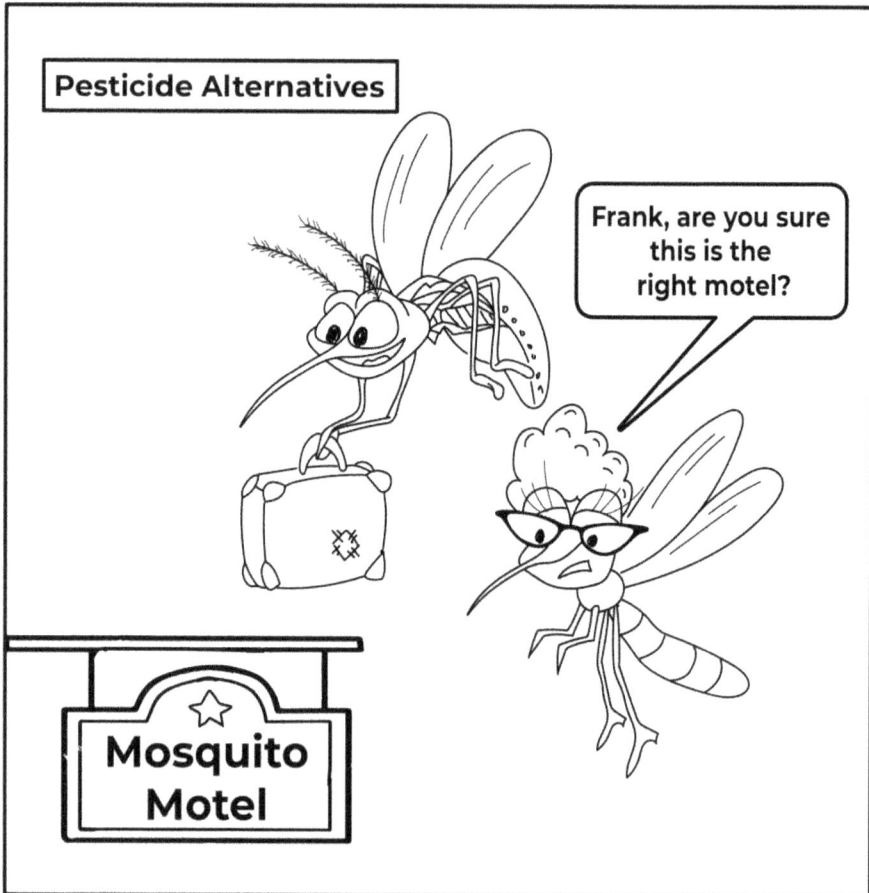

By selecting eco-friendly hardscape materials for your outdoor space, you can create a beautiful and functional landscape while minimizing your environmental footprint. These materials support your green landscaping efforts and contribute to your property's overall sustainability and health.

DR. GREG SAYS

Sunscreens and insect repellents

Let's dig into the real dirt behind sunscreens and insect repellents. I'll put on my doctor coat, and we'll explore some interesting facts about these products, their potential effects, and what's safe for you and the environment.

You might be familiar with DEET, or diethyltoluamide, as it's often the main active ingredient in many bug repellents. While DEET is remarkably effective against many pesky insects, a common misconception is that it's a high-risk toxin. However, research and the US and UK governments show that it's safe for human use when appropriately applied. Obviously, it should not be mixed into your afternoon cocktail or spread over wounds or irritated skin.

Let's turn to sunscreens. Oxybenzone and octinoxate, common ingredients in many sunscreens, are under scrutiny. Not only are they suspected of being hormone disruptors, but they're also found to cause coral bleaching. Hawaii, Key West, and several Pacific island nations have banned the sale of sunscreens containing these ingredients to protect their coral reefs.

Other ingredients to avoid include avobenzone, octisalate, and octocrylene due to their potential allergenic properties. Homosalate and octisalate are suspected of disrupting hormones and should be on your radar too.

Now onto best practices. Firstly, pick sunscreens labeled as "broad-spectrum." They protect against both UVA and UVB rays. Consider using mineral-based sunscreens with zinc oxide or titanium dioxide as active ingredients. They're safer for human health and the environment.

For insect repellents, DEET-based products remain the gold standard. However, other options like picaridin or oil of lemon eucalyptus can offer DEET-free alternatives. Always follow the product's instructions for application.

And remember, even the safest product can be harmful if misused. For sunscreens, remember to apply it 30 minutes before sun exposure and reapply at least every 2 hours or after swimming or sweating. Use just enough bug repellent to cover exposed skin and avoid over-application.

And remember what your mother said: WEAR A HAT!

Remember indoor plants!

As you focus on creating a sustainable and healthy outdoor landscape, remember to bring some green indoors. Houseplants are a fun way to brighten your day. In addition to their aesthetic appeal, indoor plants contribute to air purification, humidity regulation, and stress reduction.

Indoor plants can help improve indoor air quality by removing harmful pollutants, such as formaldehyde, benzene, and trichloroethylene, from the air. These volatile organic compounds (VOCs) are commonly found in household products and building materials and can contribute to poor indoor air quality. Plants like spider plants, snake plants, and pothos are particularly effective at removing these pollutants, improving the overall air quality in your home.

Houseplants can help regulate humidity levels by releasing moisture through a process called transpiration. This can create a more comfortable indoor environment, particularly in areas with dry indoor air. Maintaining appropriate humidity levels can also help reduce the growth of mold and dust mites, which can trigger allergies and respiratory issues.

Research has shown that having indoor plants can reduce stress levels and promote feelings of well-being. They create a more inviting and relaxing atmosphere, which can reduce anxiety and increase productivity. Caring for indoor plants can also be therapeutic and provide a sense of accomplishment as you watch them grow and thrive. For readers with relatives in a nursing home or hospital, consider gifting your loved one a plant. They'll feel better, and remarkably, it might help them live longer!

Some popular and easy-to-care-for indoor plants include:

- Spider plants: Known for their air-purifying abilities, spider plants are low-maintenance and can tolerate a range of light conditions.
- Pothos: This trailing plant is easy to care for and can thrive in low-light conditions, making it an excellent choice for rooms with limited natural light.
- Snake plants: Also known as mother-in-law's tongue, snake plants are hardy, low-maintenance, and effective at removing indoor air pollutants.
- Peace lilies: These attractive plants produce elegant white flowers and can help improve indoor air quality.
- ZZ plants: With their glossy, dark green leaves, ZZ plants are drought-tolerant and can thrive in low-light conditions.

As you work to create a sustainable and healthy outdoor landscape, remember to incorporate indoor plants into your home as well. These plants enhance the beauty of your living space and contribute to a healthier and more comfortable indoor environment.

The connection between nature and human health

The research is clear, time outdoors is good for our health.

Physical health benefits: Regular exposure to green spaces promotes a range of physical health benefits. One study published in Environmental Research demonstrated that people living in areas with more green spaces had lower levels of obesity, lower blood pressure, and lower prevalence of type 2 diabetes. Physical activity in natural environments, such as gardening or walking in a park, can improve overall health and reduce the risk of chronic diseases. Spending time in nature can also boost immune function. Research shows that exposure to natural environments can increase the production of natural killer cells, which help the body fight off infections and even cancer.

Improved cardiovascular health: Research has shown that spending time in nature is good for your heart. A study conducted in Japan found that participants who spent time in forests, a practice known as "forest bathing" or "shinrin-yoku," experienced reduced blood pressure, lower heart rates, and decreased levels of the stress hormone cortisol. These findings suggest incorporating green spaces and natural elements into your outdoor living space can improve cardiovascular fitness and reduce stress.

Gut health and the human microbiome: Exposure to nature can also improve gut health by influencing the human microbiome, the complex community of microorganisms that live in our digestive system. The human microbiome is critical in many aspects of our health, including digestion, immune function, and even mental well-being. Scientists found that exposure to natural environments can increase the diversity and resilience of our gut microbiota, which is associated with greater energy and disease resistance. By spending time in green spaces and engaging in activities like gardening, you can expose yourself to various beneficial microbes, which can help support a healthy and balanced gut microbiome.

Children's health benefits: Access to green spaces is significant for children's development and well-being. Research has shown that children with access to green spaces are more likely to engage in active play, have better motor skills, and experience lower stress and anxiety levels. Horsing around in natural environments will boost your kid's cognitive functioning and mood.

Social health benefits: Green spaces can also play a vital role in fostering social connections and community cohesion. Parks, community gardens, and other shared outdoor spaces allow people to interact, develop relationships, and engage in collaborative activities. These social connections are a vital ingredient in a satisfying life.

When we make thoughtful choices about the plants, materials, and practices we use in landscaping, we can improve our physical health, support a healthy gut microbiome, and contribute to a more sustainable and environmentally friendly world.

Interview: Linda Vater

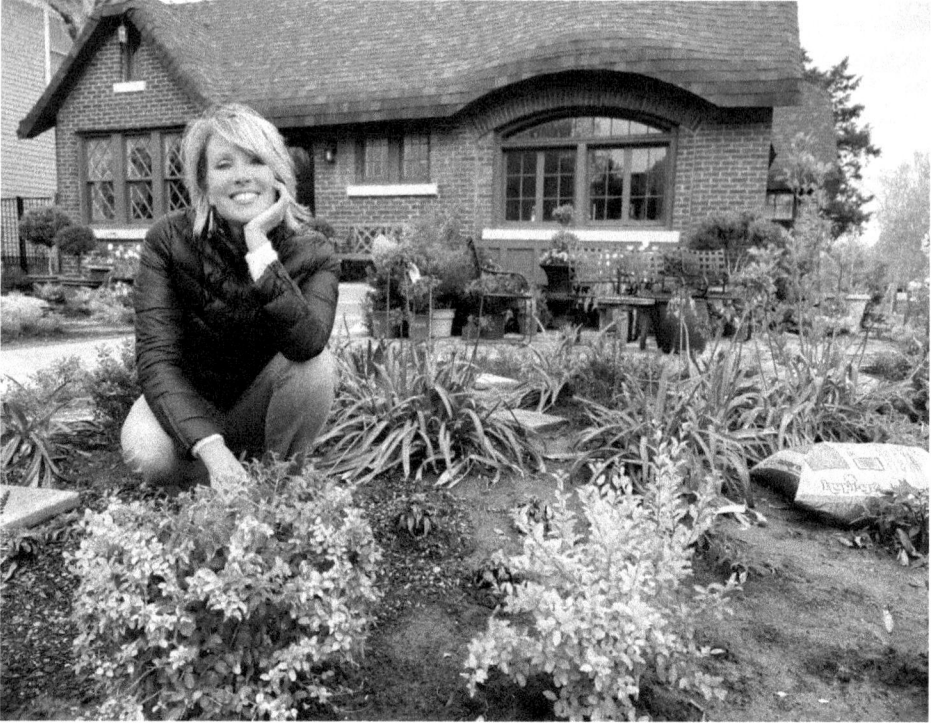

"Gardening is an act of optimism."

In a delightful interview, top influencer Linda Vater shared how personal gardening can be a simple, powerful approach to combating overwhelming global issues like loneliness, inactivity, and climate change. A passionate advocate for accessible gardening, Linda encourages people to start small, take control of their immediate environment, and make incremental changes within their reach. "I can manage this block of real estate that is my own," Linda stated, emphasizing the potential power individuals can harness by focusing on their personal spaces.

Taking control of our immediate environment can make us feel less powerless about the larger world. She cited James Clear's book, *Atomic Habits*, to illustrate the principle of starting with small, achievable actions that cumulatively build into significant change. Such changes include composting kitchen waste, reading about sustainable gardening, or employing organic pest control methods. "I can take my banana peel and throw it into the rose bush hedge. I can save my coffee grounds and use them as a soil amendment. I can start a tiny little compost pile that's just miniature in my backyard."

Linda echoes the basic premise of this book: sustainability starts at home. When we start with our own areas, we can collectively make a difference on a global scale. Linda, however, is concerned that younger people don't seem to be embracing gardening at the same rate as prior generations. She urges passionate gardeners to become evangelists for the numerous benefits gardening provides, such as protecting the environment, improved health, and enhanced quality of life.

Gardening is great for health. From physical aspects like resistance training and bone strengthening to mental benefits like improved serotonin levels and community building, gardening is a holistic wellness activity. "When I dig a hole for a shrub," Linda said, "I am getting resistance. And that resistance is making my bones stronger." Linda also stressed the role gardening can play in improving our mental well-being. "The sun just in and of itself makes you feel better," she said, emphasizing the role of nature in boosting mood and creating a sense of community. Moreover, gardening cultivates optimism and resilience as gardeners face weather events or other challenges. "It makes you feel empowered, and it makes you feel not so victimized by the planet."

Linda's philosophy is that "a garden-based life is a healthy life," with gardening as a tool to foster education, community, and stewardship of the earth. "I am just a steward here. I'm just a caretaker. It is my privilege and responsibility to care for this little parcel of earth and be a good steward as best I can."

Gardening is a powerful antidote to the recent explosion of loneliness. "One of the reasons that my channel took off is because so many people recently were just so lonely, and they just didn't feel as if they had enough people in their lives that supported them or were feeling the same things they were feeling. And the only way they could reach out was online. And so I was happy to be there for them virtually." They bonded over their love of nature and their shared quest to grow the best basket of tomatoes.

She recounted numerous personal anecdotes from her viewers who felt uplifted and comforted by her presence on their screens.

One touching story was about a woman who was so moved by Linda's videos that she decided to visit Linda's garden in Oklahoma City from Texas. Linda warmly welcomed her and listened to her heartbreaking story of dealing with a divorce and breast cancer diagnosis. "I couldn't sleep at night," she confessed to Linda. "And so I would just turn on your videos and leave them on nonstop, and you comforted me and told me I could do it. You became my friend at a time when I felt friendless."

Linda's dedication to building connections through gardening runs deep, underlined by a moving story from her childhood. She grew up in a large family with seven siblings and a widowed father. After their mother's untimely death when Linda was only five, her father often took them on evening walks around their neighborhood. Linda shared a particularly poignant memory from these walks, recalling how people would retreat into their homes as they approached, unable to confront the sorrow of her family's situation.

As an adult, being present while outside allows her to be there for others who struggle. "I think about my childhood when I am out working in the front yard and somebody stops by. Because you never know when gardening will be a lifeline for someone." She'll stop her planting and chat with anyone needing to talk. She added, "You cannot underestimate the value of a garden in forming connections." Linda's insights reminded me of recent studies suggesting that even fleeting connections with others, such as chatting with a barista at a coffee shop, can significantly contribute to happiness. She wholeheartedly agreed, saying, "And the barista felt better in return. And not only that, it's a charming way to live your life."

Near the end of our discussion, I asked Linda about making a pet-friendly yard. She suggested that gardeners make the necessary adjustments to accommodate larger pets, potentially dedicating a specific area for the pet and foregoing the idea of a perfect lawn. The key is to be informed and responsible before introducing a new plant or soil amendment to your garden. Research potential plants online to make sure they're dog-safe, for instance. Her bottom-line message was: "If you take on the responsibility of a pet, just like having a child, you become responsible at the front end—do your due diligence."

Linda is a self-taught garden designer and stylist who also writes and produces garden media for TV, magazines, Instagram, YouTube, and the web. She has lived and gardened for over thirty years in her 1935 English Tudor home before moving to her very lively "Cottage on the Hill" in Oklahoma City. Her gardens have been featured in numerous national and local magazines and have been toured more times than she can count.

Linda looks at EVERYTHING: her home, family, travel, and life's biggest questions through a gardening lens. Gardening has helped her raise two boys, be a better friend and neighbor, learn resilience, and at times saved her sanity. She says often that gardening is simultaneously one of the most joyous and frustrating things she does. Join Linda on this great adventure that is gardening.

Blog: lindavater.com

Email: info@lindavater.com

Social: @potagerblog

Interview: Dr. Wendy Hauser

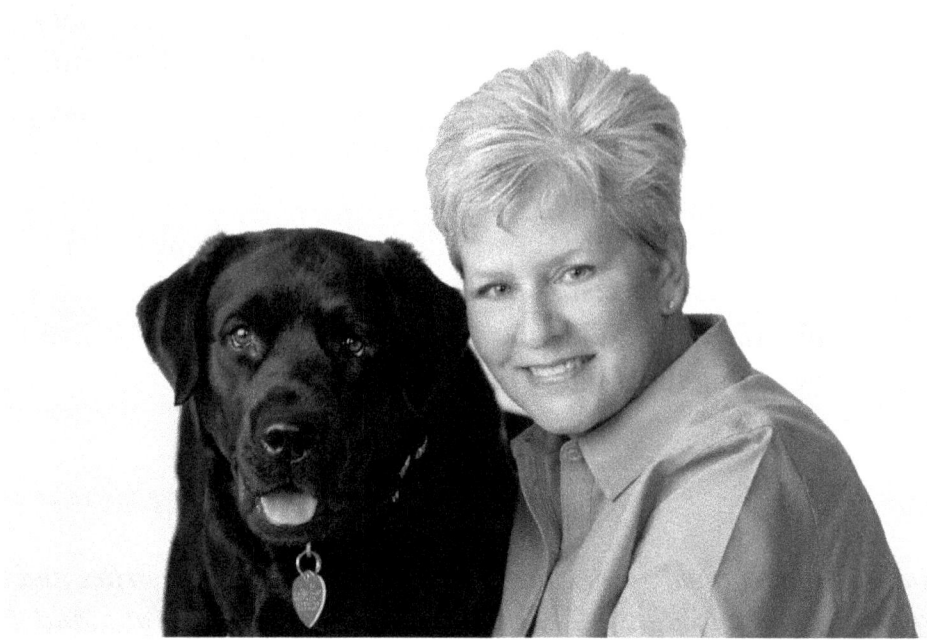

What chemicals, foods, or substances commonly in homes are most dangerous to pets?

While the dangers posed to pets are many, my patients have gotten themselves into trouble with the following household items:

- Laundry detergents and cleaning pods, like those used in washing machines and dishwashers. These are easy for dogs to ingest and cause vomiting and depression. It is possible for vomiting dogs to develop aspiration pneumonia, where the vomit accidentally enters the airways and lungs instead of being swallowed. When this occurs, it is life-threatening and requires immediate veterinary care.

One of my puppy patients knocked over a bottle of laundry detergent and was covered for hours in it before the owners returned from work. The puppy suffered severe skin inflammation from the concentrated detergent and vomiting and diarrhea from self-grooming and ingesting the laundry detergent.

- Gorilla Glue

This common wood glue expands and hardens when exposed to moisture. Dogs are exposed by either eating spilled glue or chewing on the bottles. When ingested, it expands in the stomach, forming a foreign body that requires surgical removal.

- Mouse/Rat Poison (Rodenticide) and Glue Traps

Mouse/Rat bait is designed to taste good, not only to rodents but to dogs and cats as well. Depending on the type of active ingredient in the bait, it kills the rodent by causing internal bleeding, seizures, or kidney failure. Sadly, it also affects our pets in the same way. Dogs and cats can be 'secondarily poisoned' if they ingested several rodents that have consumed the poison. Over the years, I have diagnosed many pets with rodenticide toxicity, mainly dogs that have eaten rodent bait. Most poisoned pets did not have exposure to rodent bait in their medical histories; a thorough physical examination and specific questions to the owner regarding possible exposure helped diagnose these cases.

Some homeowners prefer to use glue traps for rodent control. These, too, pose a danger to pets. Dogs, cats, and other small pets can get stuck in these traps. When trying to remove pets from traps, fur and skin are often left behind. If the pet becomes trapped while the owners aren't home, they can hurt themselves trying to escape. The most extreme case I saw as a practitioner was the pet rabbit that fractured its hind leg trying to extricate itself from the trap.

- Fiberglass Insulation

Homeowners should ensure that pets cannot access areas where fiberglass insulation is exposed. Fiberglass can cause eye, facial, and oral irritation, gastrointestinal distress, and blockages if eaten.

- Human and Pet Medications

Over-the-counter and prescription medications can be dangerous and even cause death in our pets. Pet owners should also recognize that veterinary medicines may be dangerous for other pets in the household. For example, a common anti-inflammatory for dogs, Carprofen, is toxic to cats. Additionally, because of the way it is metabolized, the active ingredient is excreted in the feces of the pet receiving the medication. There have been cases of secondary poisoning when another dog ingests these feces and is exposed to the drug. An excellent reference to learn more is the ASPCA®pro Human and Animal Medication webpage (https://www.aspcapro.org/topics-animal-health-toxicology-poison-control/human-animal-medication).

- Human Foods

Although we are all mammals, how we metabolize foods differs in different species. Owners must prevent pets from accessing certain foods. For example, xylitol is a common ingredient in natural peanut butters and sugar-free gum, yet a small amount will cause liver failure in dogs. Onions and garlic cause gastrointestinal distress and damages/destroys red blood cells in dogs and cats. Grapes and raisins can cause kidney failure in susceptible dogs. Pet owners should know what foods are safe and when to seek veterinary care if dangerous foods are ingested.

A good resource is the FDA's list of potentially dangerous items for your pet, which also highlights hazardous plants and flowers (https://www.fda.gov/animal-veterinary/animal-health-literacy/potentially-dangerous-items-your-pet).

Can poor indoor air quality (due to mold, dust, VOCs, and other chemicals) harm pets?

Poor indoor air quality is detrimental to pets, just like people. Recent studies (https://www.ncbi.nlm.nih.gov/pmc/articles/PMC7397909) have found that it can contribute to pet airway disease.

Secondhand smoke in the home places dogs, cats, and birds at higher health risks:

- Dogs have increased eye infections, allergies, and respiratory issues, including increases in lung and nasal cancer.
- Cats are at a higher risk of developing asthma, lung cancer and have double the risk of developing lymphoma (lymph node cancer).
- Birds are particularly susceptible to secondhand smoke and generally have a poorer quality of life in these environments due to skin, heart, eye, and respiratory conditions, including increases in cancer.

It is important to note that outdoor air quality also negatively impacts pets, with higher incidences of respiratory disease, including allergies, asthma, coughing, sneezing, and shortness of breath. Outdoor activities for pets should be limited when outside air quality is poor; pets should be mainly kept inside with filtered air (air conditioning and/or air filters).

What are the most common causes of traumatic injuries to household pets? How can they be avoided?

Common causes include:

Ingestion of things dogs and cats shouldn't eat, like trash that includes corn cobs and bones, as these often create intestinal blockages. Pets can also develop inflammation of the pancreas from eating fatty scraps; this is painful and can be fatal. Use pet-proof garbage containers stored behind closed doors or cabinets.

Cats are particularly prone to linear foreign bodies. If they ingest strings or thread, they get caught on the rough tongue surface and cannot be spit out. When swallowed, one end often gets caught and anchored in place. As the other end makes its way through the intestines, it creates a pleated effect, causing the intestines to bunch up. This is a surgical emergency.

Choose pet toys carefully, based on the size and level of chewing your pet exhibits. I have removed many pieces of toys from pets' stomachs and intestines. Some more interesting toys have been intact Kong toys and rubber balls, the cone forming the head of a catnip mouse, a doll shoe from a small cat's intestines, building blocks, and a rubber gasket from a toy.

- Avoid tooth damage by never giving your dog anything harder than the tooth on which to chew. One of the largest contributors to fractured teeth are bones—both real and nylon, which often cause slab fractures, where the side of the big cheek tooth is fractured and hanging on only by the gum attachment. Cow hooves can crack teeth and become embedded in the roof of the mouth.
- Dogs, cats, and rabbits will chew on electrical cords, which puts them at risk of electric shock and burns to the mouth and tongue. It is vital to pet-proof your house; plastic cord covers will help to protect pets and your electronics.
- Jumping on and off furniture can cause orthopedic issues for dogs and cats. Dog owners should train pets to use steps or ramps, particularly if they are at-risk breeds for back injuries (dachshunds, corgis, etc.). I once had a Yorkie puppy patient that broke its leg jumping off a 1" platform!

Cats live in three-dimensional worlds and need access to high places to rest and view their environment. Create stair-stepped access points, like a table to the top of a bookcase. My daughter's cat loves to sleep on top of my 4-foot filing cabinets. I have a 4-inch foam pad beside the cabinets so he lands on a cushioned surface. While he is still young, I am planning for his future joint health now!

- Safe restraint of pets

Cats are healthiest when they are kept indoors. For cats that like outside environmental enrichment, build a catio, an enclosed space that they can access through a pet door or window. This keeps the cats safe from roaming and predators like dogs, other cats, and wildlife, including birds of prey, foxes, and coyotes.

Dogs should be outside in safely fenced areas or on a leash.

What are some surprising risks to pets that owners often overlook?

The biggest risk pet owners overlook is preventing illness and disease. There is true value to the quality of life of a dog and cat when they receive regular veterinary care focused on keeping them healthy, including:

- Tip of nose to tip of tail examinations

Our pets can't tell us when they hurt or feel poorly. Thorough physical examinations include looking for obvious problems, such as lumps and bumps on the skin, and less obvious, such as spinal or abdominal pain.

- Vaccinations

Vaccinations help prevent a host of deadly and debilitating diseases. While many can be treated, they require extensive hospitalization and can have long-lasting effects.

Prevention is the key!

Preventive medications, including flea and tick prevention, heartworm prevention, and routine intestinal dewormers, will keep your pet and family safe.

- Dental Care

The most common disease in dogs and cats is periodontal disease. It is an insidious, progressive disease that impacts the quality of the pet's life, the family-pet bond, and even the pet's health. When periodontal disease progresses, the bacteria from the oral cavity are absorbed into the bloodstream and spread throughout the body to organs like the heart, liver, and kidneys. Most of all, periodontal disease hurts, and pets suffer in silence. What can pet owners do?

- Prioritize dental care:
  - Brush your pet's teeth every day. Your pet will expect it when you make it part of your daily routine. I brush my dog's teeth and my daughter's cat too every morning. Both pets follow me up the stairs and wait because it's part of their routine.
  - Look in your pet's mouth and smell its breath—it shouldn't smell 'doggy'; that means inflammation and likely periodontal disease is present.
  - Watch for changes in how your pet eats-is he chewing differently, slower, or swallowing food whole? This can indicate dental pain and the need for an oral examination at the veterinary practice.
  - When advised, have your pet's teeth professionally cleaned under anesthesia. Even though I am diligent with the dog and cat's dental health, they need professional cleanings and x-rays, just like me!
- Weight control

Obesity is the second most common disease in dogs and cats. According to studies, it has worsened in the past decade, with a 108% increase in dogs diagnosed as overweight and obese. The increase in cats was even greater, at 114%.

Not only is this dangerous to the health and well-being of the pet, but it also costs owners more. Owners of overweight dogs spend 17% more on healthcare costs and nearly 25% more on medications due to obesity-related diseases than owners of optimal-weight dogs. Cat owners with overweight cats paid 36% more on diagnostics than those whose cats were svelte.

Please talk with your vet to learn how to identify a healthy weight for your pet and the steps to achieve and maintain that weight. A great resource for self-education is found at the Association for Pet Obesity Prevention (https://www.petobesityprevention.org/).

What are common outdoor dangers to household pets, i.e., poisonous plants, pesticides, landscape design, fences, predators, etc.?

There are so many plants, both ornamental and vegetable, that are pleasing to us but harmful to our pets. Readers should refer to the extensive list at the ASPCA® Poisonous Plants site (https://www.aspca.org/pet-care/animal-poison-control/toxic-and-non-toxic-plants).

What should owners consider when leaving dogs outside, especially unsupervised?

- What type of collar is on your pet?

I have lost two different patients to hanging. They were left outside unattended with choke chain collars, which tragically became hooked on fences, and the pets suffocated. I counsel clients to use flat buckle collars for everyday use and use martingales or choke collars only when walking the dog. Cats should also wear collars; they should be of breakaway design so the cat can escape if it gets caught under furniture, etc. Both cats and dogs should have identification tags on collars, and, as dictated by local ordinances, rabies vaccination tags. When placing tags on a cat collar, I prefer the flat tag that fits onto the collar itself, so nothing is dangling.

- Wildlife can pose risks to pets.

Small dogs and cats are at risk of being prey for coyotes, foxes, and birds of prey. They should never be left unattended outside. I have treated dogs attacked by owls and coyotes. While most have survived, not all have; it is heartbreaking for their families. Pet owners should be cautious around the larger wildlife species, such as deer, elk, and moose, especially when the wildlife has babies. They will attack and seriously hurt the dogs by kicking, goring, or stamping them. Pet owners should keep dogs leashed when these wildlife are present and give them a wide berth.

Is it true that certain breeds of pet dogs are more dangerous to humans?

I disagree with this statement; I think it is important to select a breed that fits the family's needs. Owners should consider the following:

- What lifestyle and activities do they want to do with the dog?
- Some breeds of dogs are better suited for outdoor activities such as hiking and camping, while others are better around-the-block companions.
- What level of grooming do they want to commit to?
- Some breeds require frequent and often professional grooming, while others are lower maintenance, wash-and-wear dogs.
- What is the family composition, humans and other animals?

If young children are in the household, a 'sturdier' dog might be better than a teacup Poodle or Yorkshire Terrier. A sturdier dog might be better if larger dogs are in the home.

- How much does the owner plan to spend on veterinary care?

Some breeds have a higher incidence of genetic and inherited disorders. The most popular breed, the French Bulldog, has been selectively bred to have an extremely flat face contributing to respiratory problems necessitating pro-active surgical modification while puppies, which costs thousands of dollars. As a former owner of a Cavalier King Charles Spaniel, I can attest to how marvelous they are. Unfortunately, these dogs have neurologic and heart disease due to a very narrow ancestry.

Owning these breeds is expensive; pet owners should expect to spend significantly more on these dogs than other breeds. While pet insurance is helpful, due to the costly claims filed within these breeds, the monthly premiums are often higher and pre-existing conditions are usually not covered.

How can an owner know what dog is best for them?

- Several organizations, like the AKC, have breed selector tools (https://www.akc.org/breed-selector-tool/). I recommend a book, *Paws to Consider*, by Brian Kilcommons, to my clients when deciding what breed best fits their family.
- Mixed-breed dogs from shelters and rescues make excellent pets. Most reputable shelters have adoption counselors to help pet owners find their perfect match.
- Educate yourself about the most common inherited diseases (https://www.akc.org/dog-breeds/) for the breed you select, and if purchasing from a breeder, be sure to ask about screening tests for these diseases. Asking the right questions will help to reduce the risk of heartache later.

How does pet insurance work? What sorts of problems does it cover? What types and ages of animals are typically covered?

Pet insurance is a financial tool that helps pet owners share the risk of pet ownership with the insurer. It is not an investment tool; an owner's goal should be never to need it because that means your pet remains healthy. It's a safety net, so the client has help paying for eligible veterinary care if unexpected accidents or illnesses happen, taking the stress out of decision-making.

Unlike human health insurance, it is a property insurance product, and the insurance relationship is between the pet owner and the insurance company. There are no networks; most pet insurance companies allow pet owners to take their pet to any licensed veterinarian in the US, and depending on the company, in Canada.

These policies cover care in general, emergency, and specialty veterinary facilities.

There are different types of policies, including accident and illness, or accident only. Some providers also offer preventive care coverage as an add-on option for an additional cost. Most pet insurance plans do not cover pre-existing conditions, which is very different from human health insurance coverage. Because of this, it makes sense to get coverage before any conditions develop or at least understand that some existing conditions could be excluded from coverage.

Depending upon the pet insurance plan and company, owners can often choose the following:

- The annual coverage level is the maximum amount they can get reimbursed in one year.
- The deductible is the amount paid out of pocket before getting reimbursed. Some companies have annual deductibles, and others are condition-specific deductibles. This impacts the out-of-pocket expense and is something to understand before enrolling in a policy.
- The reimbursement percentage is how much will be paid for eligible expenses.

These three factors can impact the monthly policy premium. For example, the monthly premium payment is typically lower when there is a smaller annual coverage limit, a higher deductible, and a lower reimbursement percentage. Pet owners should determine how much out-of-pocket expenses they can afford when choosing their policy limits, bearing in mind that the cost of veterinary care continues to increase.

Most providers cover dogs and cats; some providers cover horses and exotic pets, such as reptiles and birds. Age eligibility may vary depending on the policy.

For what families or situations would you particularly recommend pet insurance?

I believe that pet insurance is a necessity, not a luxury. Due to the increasing costs of providing veterinary care, the cost to owners is also increasing. I have never met a pet owner that didn't want what's best for their pet. However, I have met many who couldn't afford the needed care, which is heartbreaking for the owner, the veterinary team, the veterinarian, and the pet.

I recommend that owners ask their veterinarians about the anticipated lifetime cost of care for their pet, the common health problems with this breed, and how much it can cost to address these likely issues. Owners should then assess how much they can pay out of pocket and strategize how to provide unexpected care BEFORE it's needed. One of the tools that can help pet owners is pet insurance. Others include wellness plans to help pay for preventive care and third-party options like dedicated pet credit cards.

Pet insurance is becoming a common employee benefit, so pet owners should check with their employers to see if it is offered. Often, these plans are competitively priced compared to an open market plan.

How can people evaluate and choose the right type of pet insurance for their needs?

Pet owners should read the sample policy plans on each provider's website to ensure the coverage meets their needs. Additionally, most providers have customer care teams that can answer questions.

Pet owners should also check reviews; a good site for this is Trustpilot (https://www.trustpilot.com/categories/pet_insurance_company). Check the BBB ratings and the AM Best insurance ratings as well.

Wendy Hauser, DVM, is the founder of Peak Veterinary Consulting and has practiced for 30+ years as an associate, practice owner, and relief veterinarian. She has worked in the animal health industry as a pet health insurance executive and a technical services veterinarian.

Dr. Hauser, passionate about education and innovation, consults with industry partners (emerging and established) and individual veterinary hospitals. She is a regular presenter at veterinary conferences, facilitating workshops on hospital culture, associate development, leadership, client relations, and operations. Frequently published, she co-authors "The Veterinarian's Guide to Healthy Pet Plans."

Dr. Hauser lives in the Denver Metro area with her husband, Edmond, and their black Lab, Oliver. She has two grown children; her son is a consultant in the energy field and lives in the Denver Metro area. Her daughter graduated from medical school and is in the first year of an OB-GYN residency.

Contact information:

https://peakveterinaryconsulting.com/

linkedin.com/in/wendyhauserdvm

CHAPTER 14

Renewable Energy, Micromobility, and the Future

Welcome to Greener Grove, home to the avant-garde and eco-conscious Clark family. The air is clean, the birds are singing, and the sun shines just a bit brighter. With their solar-powered home and penchant for zipping around on micromobility devices, the Clarks found a way to make sustainability fun.

On any given day, you might find Mr. Clark whipping up a mean avocado toast in the kitchen, powered by energy-efficient appliances humming away on the sun's energy. Meanwhile, Mrs. Clark bags lunches for the kids, wrapping sandwiches in reusable beeswax wrappers as she sings her favorite 80s power ballads. Little Tommy and Susie grab their lunches and zip outside, eager to hop on their electric scooters for the ride to school.

As the Clarks go about their day, their home soaks up the warm sunshine, efficiently converting it into electricity through the sleek solar panels perched on their roof. The family car, a snazzy electric vehicle manufactured in Georgia, waits impatiently in the driveway, ready for its next emission-free adventure.

The Clarks' passion for sustainable living extends beyond their home as they enthusiastically embrace the world of micromobility. Every evening, you'll find them cruising through the neighborhood on their electric scooters or bikes, laughing as they zoom past the more traditional, gas-guzzling cars. The family's favorite weekend activity? Racing each other in electric go-karts, of course!

Through their commitment to green living, the Clarks have discovered that being eco-conscious doesn't mean sacrificing adventure or convenience. Their sustainable choices have enriched their lives and brought them closer together.

They enjoy lower utility bills, superior indoor air quality, and a strong sense of community with their like-minded neighbors in Greener Grove. With their solar-powered home and love for micromobility, the Clarks are living proof that going green can be both enjoyable and practical.

Solar Power and Batteries

Solar power is a critical component of the Clark's sustainable lifestyle. But what are the pros and cons of solar energy? Let's dive in and explore the advantages and disadvantages of this renewable energy source.

Pros:

1. Renewable and abundant: Solar energy is renewable, meaning it won't run out, unlike fossil fuels. The sun provides an almost limitless supply of energy that can be harnessed by solar panels, offering a sustainable solution for meeting our energy needs as the global population continues to grow.

2. Reduces electricity bills: Solar energy can significantly reduce or eliminate electricity bills. By generating their power, families like the Clarks can save money on their monthly expenses and even earn credits for the excess energy they feed back into the grid.

3. Low maintenance: Solar panels require little maintenance, making them an attractive option for busy families like the Clarks. Occasional cleaning and inspection are typically all that's needed, and many solar panel manufacturers offer long-term warranties, giving homeowners peace of mind.

4. Environmentally friendly: Solar energy produces no greenhouse gas emissions or air pollution, contributing to cleaner air and a healthier environment. Families can reduce their carbon footprint by choosing solar power and help combat climate change.

5. Energy independence: With solar power, homeowners can reduce their reliance on the grid and enjoy greater energy independence. They'll sure appreciate owning their energy source next time the county's power grid goes down!

6. Tax credits and incentives may be available (see below).

Cons:

1. Intermittent: Solar energy depends on sunlight, so it's unavailable at night or during cloudy days. This is why the Clarks have invested in a battery system to store excess energy for later use. However, the cost of battery storage can be prohibitive for some homeowners.

2. High upfront costs: Solar panel installation can be expensive, with the average price ranging from $15,000 to $25,000 before incentives. However, government programs and financing options can help offset these costs, and the long-term savings often outweigh the initial investment.

3. Space requirements: Solar panels need sufficient space for installation, which may be an issue for those with limited roof space or living in densely populated areas. Ground-

mounted systems are an alternative but may require even more space and additional permits. Care must be taken when installing solar panels on older roofs.

4. Aesthetics: Some people may find the appearance of solar panels unattractive. However, technological advances have led to the development of solar shingles and other more visually appealing options, which can blend seamlessly with traditional roofing materials.

5. Environmental impact: Manufacturing solar panels isn't easy. Rare earth elements and other difficult-to-obtain materials are often necessary for solar panels. Moreover, many solar panels are challenging to recycle. Therefore, solar panels might do the environment more harm than good in areas with little sunlight.

6. Geographic limitations: Cloudy areas may not generate enough power to make the investment worthwhile.

As you can imagine, solar panels work best in sunny places. If you live in a cold, cloudy area, it's doubtful that you'll benefit from these gizmos. Each state has vastly different energy policies and financial incentives, influencing your economic calculus when determining whether to go solar.

Before we continue, let's take a quick look at Net Metering

Net metering is a billing arrangement that allows homeowners with solar power systems to receive credit for any excess electricity they generate and feed back into the grid. In essence, it enables the electric meter to run forwards and backward, measuring the difference between the electricity consumed from the grid and the electricity generated by the solar panels.

When a solar power system produces more electricity than the household needs, the excess energy is returned to the utility grid. With net metering, homeowners receive a credit on their electric bill for this returned energy at the same rate they would pay for electricity from the grid. When solar panels produce less electricity than the household needs, homeowners can use these credits to offset their energy consumption from the grid, effectively lowering their electricity bills.

Net metering encourages the adoption of renewable energy sources like solar power by providing financial incentives for homeowners and promoting energy independence. It also benefits the utility grid by supplying clean, renewable energy during peak demand periods, reducing the need for additional power plants, and minimizing the environmental impact of electricity generation.

Top 5 Best States for Home Solar

1. California: With abundant sunshine and strong solar incentives, California is a leader in solar energy adoption. The state's policies, such as the California Solar Initiative, make it easier for homeowners to invest in solar energy and reap the benefits.
2. Arizona: The state's sunny climate and net metering policies make it an attractive place for solar installations. Arizona also offers solar equipment and installation tax credits, which help reduce the upfront costs of going solar.
3. New Jersey: Despite its relatively small size, New Jersey boasts generous solar incentives and a robust solar market. The state's Solar Renewable Energy Certificate (SREC) program allows homeowners to earn money for the solar energy they generate.
4. Massachusetts: Massachusetts offers numerous financial incentives, such as the Solar Massachusetts Renewable Target (SMART) program, and a solar-friendly regulatory environment, making it an appealing destination for those looking to harness solar power.

5. Colorado: The Centennial State has a thriving solar industry, thanks to its abundant sunshine, strong net metering policies, and state tax credits for solar installations.

Toughest 5 States for Home Solar

1. Mississippi: Mississippi ranks low in solar adoption due to its lack of solar incentives and unfavorable net metering policies.
2. South Dakota: With minimal state incentives and a cooler, cloudier climate, South Dakota's solar market is underdeveloped compared to other states.
3. Alaska: Although Alaska offers some solar rebates, the state's short daylight hours during winter and limited solar resources make it a challenging environment for homeowners.
4. West Virginia: West Virginia's coal-centric energy policies and minimal solar incentives have resulted in a sluggish solar market within the state.
5. Oklahoma: Despite its relatively sunny climate, Oklahoma's solar market suffers from unfavorable net metering policies and a lack of state incentives.

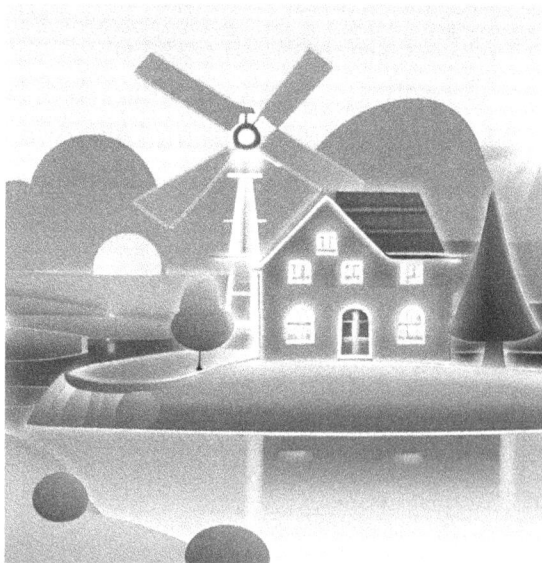

Lease vs. Buy Solar Panels

Deciding whether to lease or buy solar panels can be tricky. Here are some key points to consider:

Leasing:

1. Lower upfront costs: Leasing solar panels typically requires little to no money down, making it an attractive option for those with limited upfront capital.
2. Maintenance included: The leasing company is responsible for maintenance and repairs, which can be a plus for homeowners who prefer to avoid dealing with these responsibilities.
3. No ownership: When you lease solar panels, you don't own the system, meaning you may miss out on some financial benefits, such as tax credits and increased property value.

Buying:

1. Long-term savings: Buying solar panels can lead to sizable long-term savings. In a suitable locale, you'll benefit from reduced electricity bills and potential income from selling excess energy back to the grid.
2. Tax credits and incentives: Homeowners who purchase solar panels are eligible for federal and state tax credits, as well as other incentives, which can significantly reduce the cost of the system.
3. Increased property value: Studies have shown that solar panels can increase the value of a home, making it a wise investment for homeowners planning to sell their property in the future.

With leased and purchased panels, be careful about what debt you attach to your property. Selling your home may be more challenging if your buyer has to assume your loan or lease.

Ultimately, the decision to lease or buy solar panels depends on your financial situation, long-term plans, and personal preferences. Be sure to secure quotes from multiple installers to see if you can score a sweet deal.

Let's shift our focus to another important aspect of green home renovations: the choice between natural gas and electricity for home use.

Natural gas and electricity each have their advantages and disadvantages when it comes to powering homes. Understanding these pros and cons can help you decide which energy source best fits your needs.

Natural gas is known for its efficiency and cost-effectiveness. It's a highly reliable energy source that you can use for heating, cooking, and even generating electricity. According to the EIA, natural gas is the most common heating fuel in the United States. Many homeowners prefer it due to its relatively lower cost than electricity. Additionally, natural gas appliances are quite energy-efficient, reducing energy bills.

Some chefs prefer cooking with natural gas; a fancy gas-powered stove might be a powerful perk when you sell your home.

One quick aside about the benefit of natural gas for power generation. Back in my Texas days, we weathered a terrible ice storm that shut down the power grid. For days, we had no electricity, internet, or HEAT. It was 19 degrees outside and not much warmer inside. We are all freezing! Those icy days didn't get us off on the right foot (paw?) with our recently adopted puppy.

Our neighbors, it turns out, were smarter than we were. Right before the storm, they invested in a power generator that connected directly to the gas line. While we were huddled up in PJs under woolen blankets in the dark, they were sipping cocktails and riding out the weather in style.

Of course, you can potentially enjoy the same peace of mind with a powerful home battery that stores your solar energy. I mention this cautionary tale as food for thought when deciding how best to secure your electricity supply in an emergency.

There are downsides to using natural gas. Natural gas extraction, production, and transportation contribute to greenhouse gas emissions, which can negatively poison the environment. Furthermore, natural gas leaks can pose safety hazards, increasing the risk of fires or explosions in homes.

Burning natural gas may harm indoor air quality by releasing toxins, including nitrogen dioxide and ultrafine particulate matter. There's some evidence that gas stoves (via these toxic byproducts) may increase the risk of childhood asthma and other diseases.

Electricity may offer a more versatile and environmentally friendly option. By powering a home with electricity, homeowners can easily transition to renewable energy sources, such as solar or wind, which can reduce their carbon footprint and help combat climate change. Moreover, electric appliances are generally safer than their gas counterparts, as there are no combustion-related risks or leaks to worry about.

Unfortunately, electricity can be more expensive than natural gas, depending on the region and utility rates. Furthermore, electricity production often relies on non-renewable resources, such as coal, which can also contribute to greenhouse gas emissions. Thankfully, we're trending towards greener electric generation, mitigating this problem.

In summary, both natural gas and electricity have their own unique set of advantages and drawbacks. Homeowners should carefully consider cost, environmental impact, and safety when deciding which energy source best fits their needs.

As we continue exploring the various aspects of green home renovations, let's delve into electric vehicles (EVs) and home charging solutions.

With the growing popularity of EVs, many homeowners are looking to install EV chargers in their homes. Let's review the various charging options.

There are three main types of EV chargers, classified as Level 1, Level 2, and DC fast charging. Level 1 chargers are the most basic, using a standard 120-volt outlet and providing a slow charge, typically adding about 4 to 5 miles of range per hour. While these chargers don't require special installation, their slow charging speed may not be sufficient for some users.

Level 2 chargers offer a faster charging option, using a 240-volt outlet and adding 10 to 60 miles of range per hour. This is a more practical choice for many EV owners. However, Level 2 chargers often require professional installation, which can add to the overall cost.

As an aside, I hope that more condos, apartment complexes, and multifamily communities will install Level 2 chargers. As it stands, EV ownership is typically restricted to homeowners due to the lack of public overnight charging stations. Adding charging stations to multifamily dwellings will make EVs accessible to more communities. To the builders and investors reading this book, I hope you consider adding charging stations to your multifamily properties regardless of location. You'll do a good deed by making EV access more equitable, and your tenants will love you!

And while we're on the topic, if you are a builder or investor reading this book, I hope you will consider installing solar panels on your multiunit properties. If you're in a sunny location, the panels will save your tenants a bundle on utility bills - making your property the hot spot in town.

DC fast chargers provide the quickest charging speeds, replenishing 60 to 80 miles of range in just 20 minutes. While this may sound ideal, DC fast chargers are typically in public charging stations. They are rarely in residential settings due to their high cost and substantial power requirements. If you have one in your condo, you hit a home run.

When considering whether to install an EV charger in your home or condo, weighing the pros and cons is essential. A home charger offers convenience and time savings, as you can charge your EV overnight or whenever you park at home. Additionally, home charging can be more cost-effective than relying on public charging stations, especially if you can take advantage of off-peak electricity rates.

On the downside, a Level 2 charger requires an upfront investment for both the charger and the professional installation. Furthermore, not all homes or condos have the necessary electrical infrastructure to support a Level 2 charger, which may require costly upgrades.

Micromobility

As the world continues to embrace cleaner transportation solutions, micromobility is emerging as an increasingly popular option. Micromobility refers to small, lightweight electric vehicles, such as e-scooters and golf carts, for short trips in urban environments.

E-scooters have gained significant traction in recent years, offering a convenient, eco-friendly, and often cost-effective mode of short-distance transportation. They have become trendy in densely populated cities, where they help alleviate traffic congestion and reduce air pollution. A study conducted in Paris found that e-scooters are safe and increasingly replacing car use, making them an attractive alternative for city dwellers.

Golf carts, too, are finding a new purpose in urban settings, thanks to their compact size and electric powertrains. In places like Peachtree City, Georgia, golf carts have become a primary mode of transportation. Residents love zipping down the city's extensive network of cart paths. Talk about a modern town!

While micromobility offers numerous benefits, it's essential to recognize that these vehicles also have drawbacks. For instance, e-scooters have faced criticism over safety concerns and fire risks. Their overall environmental impact depends on factors such as battery manufacturing and disposal processes. There is some debate about the value of e-scooter rentals in cities. However, there is no doubt that you're doing the planet a solid when you hop in your e-scooter to visit the neighbor down the block rather than firing up your SUV (as long as your garage doesn't catch fire!). If you decide to get an electric scooter, be sure to do your research and pick a reputable brand.

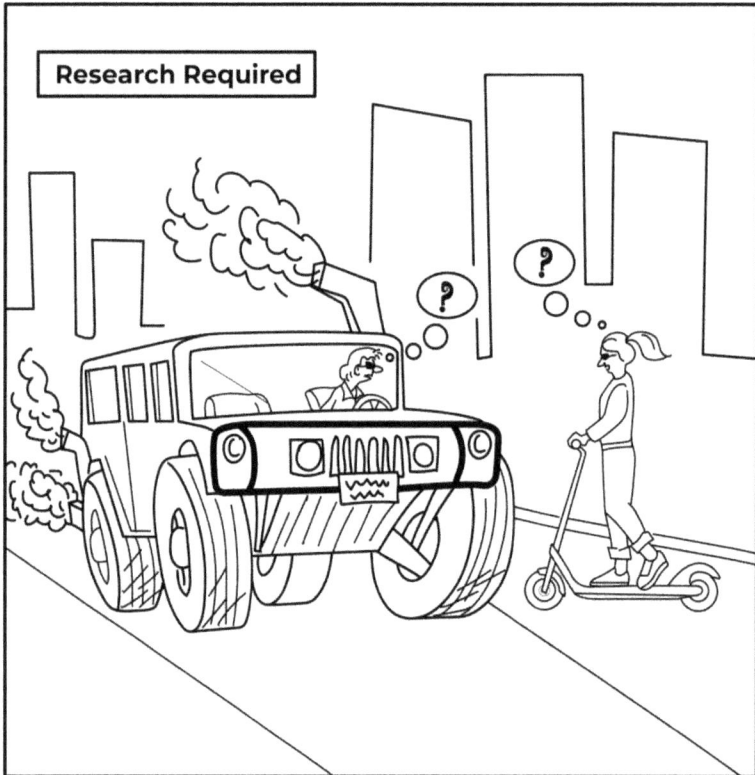

© Dr. Greg. LLC 2023

As you consider incorporating sustainable practices into your home renovations, understanding the various green building certifications available is essential. These certifications provide a framework for designing, constructing, and maintaining environmentally friendly, energy-efficient homes. They also offer guidelines for assessing a home's environmental impact and performance. Some popular green building certifications include LEED for Homes, the National Green Building Standard®, ENERGY STAR, and Passive House.

LEED (Leadership in Energy and Environmental Design) for Homes is a widely recognized green building certification program developed by the U.S. Green Building Council (USGBC). LEED-certified homes are designed and built to be resource-efficient, using less water and energy. They generate fewer greenhouse gas emissions compared to traditional homes. LEED certification also considers factors such as indoor air quality, access to public transportation, and use of sustainable materials. There are various levels of LEED certification (Certified, Silver, Gold, and Platinum), which are determined based on a point system that evaluates a home's environmental performance across several categories.

The National Green Building Standard® (NGBS) is another green home certification program developed by the National Association of Home Builders (NAHB) and the International Code Council (ICC). The NGBS provides a flexible, rigorous, and affordable path for builders and developers to achieve green certification for their projects. Like LEED, the NGBS certification includes several levels (Bronze, Silver, Gold, and Emerald) based on the home's performance. It encompasses various aspects of green building, such as energy efficiency, water conservation, and indoor air quality.

ENERGY STAR is a well-known certification program focused on energy efficiency. Homes that earn the ENERGY STAR label must meet strict guidelines set by the US Environmental Protection Agency (EPA) for energy efficiency, which can result in significant energy savings and reduced greenhouse gas emissions. ENERGY STAR-certified homes often include high-performance windows, efficient heating and cooling systems, and comprehensive air sealing to minimize drafts.

Passive House is an international building standard that focuses on ultra-energy-efficient building design. Passive House-certified buildings require very little energy for heating and cooling, making them up to 90% more energy-efficient than conventional buildings. Strategies such as super-insulation, airtight construction, high-performance windows, and heat recovery ventilation systems that provide fresh air while minimizing energy loss yield tremendous efficiency.

Green building certifications offer numerous benefits for homeowners, including reduced energy and water consumption, improved indoor air quality, increased property values, and potential access to financial incentives and tax credits. Furthermore, they are a valuable guide for homeowners making informed decisions about eco-friendly home renovations. Plus, you'll make bank when you sell your certified house!

As the world moves toward a more sustainable future, numerous emerging trends and technologies shape how we power our homes. Here are ten of the most notable home energy trends to watch for:

1. Solar roof tiles: Solar shingles or tiles are an innovative solution that allows homeowners to generate clean energy without installing traditional solar panels. These shingles integrate seamlessly with existing roof materials, providing a more aesthetically pleasing option for solar power generation.

2. Smart home energy management: Advanced home energy management systems use real-time data and automation to optimize energy usage, helping homeowners save money and reduce their environmental impact. These systems often incorporate intelligent thermostats, lighting controls, and appliances that can be remotely monitored and controlled.

3. Battery storage systems: As more homeowners adopt renewable energy sources like solar and wind, energy

storage solutions like home battery systems are becoming increasingly popular. These systems store excess energy generated during peak production periods and allow for its use during higher demand or low renewable energy generation. Powerful batters reduce reliance on grid electricity, lower energy costs, and improve resilience during power outages. I could have used one of these in Texas!

4. Electric vehicle (EV) charging: With the growing popularity of electric cars, many homeowners are installing EV charging stations to conveniently and efficiently recharge their vehicles. This trend will likely continue as EV adoption increases and more vehicle models become available. Chargers will also boost your home's resale value, as many buyers expect to find them in the garage.

5. Home energy audits: Homeowners are becoming more proactive in assessing their home's energy efficiency and identifying areas for improvement. Home energy audits, which involve a professional evaluation of a home's energy usage, insulation, heating and cooling systems, and other factors, can help pinpoint inefficiencies and suggest actionable steps for reducing energy consumption. For more information, see the chapter on home energy audits.

6. Energy-efficient windows: High-performance windows minimize heat transfer, keeping homes cooler in the summer and warmer in the winter. This can result in significant energy savings and improved comfort. Energy-efficient windows often feature low-emissivity coatings, double or triple glazing, and insulated frames. Triple-pane and modern materials are reshaping how we view windows.

7. Geothermal heating and cooling: Geothermal systems tap into the earth's stable temperature to provide efficient heating and cooling for homes. These systems can be a more environmentally friendly alternative to traditional

heating and cooling methods, as they use significantly less energy and produce fewer greenhouse gas emissions.

8. Green roofs and walls: Green roofs and walls, which involve the integration of plants and vegetation on building surfaces, offer numerous benefits, including improved insulation, stormwater management, and increased biodiversity. These living structures can also help combat the urban heat island effect, reducing the need for air conditioning and lowering energy consumption. When possible, be sure to choose native plants that attract pollinators.

9. Heat pumps: Heat pumps are a highly efficient and versatile heating and cooling solution that can provide heating and cooling using a single system. They work by transferring heat between indoor and outdoor environments rather than generating it directly, making them more energy-efficient than traditional furnaces and air conditioners.

10. Community Solar Associations: While not technically a *technology*, Community Solar Associations are cooperative arrangements that allow multiple participants to share the benefits of a solar power installation. In this setup, a solar system is installed in a shared location, and the energy it produces is distributed among the participants, typically as credits on their electricity bills. This arrangement allows individuals who cannot or prefer not to install solar panels on their own property to still benefit from renewable energy. These associations promote environmental sustainability while providing a financially accessible way for people to use clean energy. They're quite common in Europe and are finding their way into the US.

By staying informed about these emerging trends and technologies, homeowners can make more eco-friendly choices when renovating or building their homes. Together, we can make all our towns as eco-friendly as Greener Grove!

DR. GREG SAYS

Get your kids outside

Your child is an adventurer, a pint-sized explorer setting foot into a world of endless possibilities. That's what stepping outside can be like for your little ones. The great outdoors is more than just open space—it's a vast, real-life playground that packs a powerful punch for their well-being. So, strap on their tiny hiking boots, and let's explore the powerful mental and physical health benefits of playing outside.

1. It Fosters Physical Fitness: Research from Children's Hospital of Philadelphia shows that outdoor play is one of the best ways to keep kids physically fit. Whether running, climbing, or participating in a sport, kids strengthen their muscles, improve their coordination, and maintain a healthy weight when playing outside. Plus, these activities are just plain fun!

2. It Promotes Healthy Vision: Harvard Health notes that sunlight exposure is good for children's eyes. It helps to prevent the development of nearsightedness, or myopia, a common condition where faraway objects appear blurry. So, when kids look up from their screens and gaze out at nature, they're doing their eyes a favor.

3. It Encourages Social Skills: The American Academy of Pediatrics (AAP) suggests that outdoor play can improve kids' social abilities. Children learn how to work together, solve problems, and communicate when they play outside. This can help them form stronger relationships and boost their self-confidence.

4. It Supports Cognitive and Emotional Development: Playing outside also improves children's health in ways that are harder to see but just as important. The Early Childhood Learning and Knowledge Center states that outdoor play can enhance children's cognitive growth and emotional well-being. Nature's randomness prompts them to think creatively and adapt, while the freedom and space to explore can reduce stress and promote happiness.

5. It Offers a Hands-On Way to Learn About Nature: Gardening is a fantastic outdoor activity for children. As *Psychology Today* points out, gardening provides physical exercise and instills an appreciation for nature, teaches responsibility, and offers lessons in science. Plus, when children see their hard work bloom into beautiful flowers or delicious fruits or vegetables, they learn the power of perseverance.

6. It Improves Immunity through Microbiome Exposure: Believe it or not, dirt is good for kids. Numerous studies suggest that exposure to diverse microbes in natural environments, such as soil, can bolster the immune system. This process is often referred to as the "hygiene hypothesis." The idea is that exposure to various bacteria and other microorganisms in early life can "train" the immune system to fight off disease more effectively. Certain soil bacteria seem to stimulate the production of serotonin, a mood-regulating hormone, contributing to emotional well-being. When children dig in the dirt, they have fun and build healthier, more resilient bodies.

I love taking my daughters to the local nursery. They get to choose their favorite plants and shrubs. We cross-check an app to ensure they're easy to grow, non-toxic to dogs, and play well with our Georgia climate. Once we're home, they plant everything in our raised garden bed. As a family, we have fun every morning, checking out our colorful blooms.

Mother Nature is the ultimate pediatrician. So, let's take the prescription to heart: more outdoor play, more often!

CHAPTER 15

Are Green Remodels Worth It?

In 2020, I published my best-selling book, *Why Doctors Skip Breakfast: Wellness Tips to Reverse Aging, Treat Depression, and Get a Good Night's Sleep*. It helped countless individuals discover ways to live longer, stay young, and find a sense of wellness in their everyday lives. But just as medical knowledge evolves, so does the world of green home renovations.

I must admit that I'm embarrassed by some of my medical beliefs from way back in the day.

Quick confession. Remember some time ago when we thought fat was the only dietary poison? We believed we'd be all good if we could just avoid the oil. So, as a kid, I took this concept a bit too far. I don't know if y'all remember Reduced Fat Oreos. Well, I loved those things - I ate 'em by the case. But hey, I told myself, they're all good because they have 35% less fat.

Well, I'm still trying to burn off those calories now as an adult.

The point is, when it comes to making our homes more eco-friendly, we need to stay informed and open-minded. Green technology is like medicine—both constantly change, and there's always something new to learn. In this chapter, we'll dive into the world of sustainable home remodels and explore whether they're worth the investment. So, grab your tool belt, put on your doctor's coat, and let's get started!

Before we start, let's take a moment to acknowledge that this information is subject to change. As technology advances, costs fluctuate, new trends emerge, and the specifics of what makes a remodel eco-friendly and cost-effective will evolve. Additionally, factors like climate and location can impact the effectiveness and savings of certain upgrades.

While I strive to provide accurate and up-to-date information, it's essential that you research and consult with professionals to ensure you make the best decisions for your unique situation and consider all the options available. Review the IRS website and consult with a tax professional to ensure you make the best decisions for your situation.

With that out of the way, let's discuss some incentives that can make green home remodels even more appealing.

Local, state, and federal incentives

One of the great things about going green with your home renovations is that financial incentives are often available at the local, state, and federal levels. While I am not an accountant or financial advisor, I can point you toward some resources to help you find the most current information on these incentives.

On the federal level, the IRS offers various tax credits for energy-efficient home improvements. One significant incentive is the Residential Renewable Energy Tax Credit, which covers solar energy systems, wind turbines, and geothermal heat pumps. This credit allows homeowners to claim up to 26% of the cost of installing these systems as a tax credit, with no upper limit. The rebate percentage will decrease to 22%, and the credit is set to expire by 2024. Review the IRS guidelines and consult a tax professional to ensure eligibility.

Another federal tax incentive is the Nonbusiness Energy Property Credit, which provides a credit for energy-saving improvements like insulation, energy-efficient windows, and certain heating and cooling systems. This credit has a lifetime cap of $500 with specific limits.

The Energy Efficient Home Credit provides a tax credit for contractors building energy-efficient homes, which can result in more affordable green housing options for consumers.

The Department of Energy (DOE) also offers various resources and programs to support energy efficiency and renewable energy in homes. The Solar Rooftop Potential tool can help you assess the viability of solar panels, and Energy.gov provides a cost calculator to estimate potential savings from solar installations.

State and local incentives vary depending on location, but many states offer tax credits, rebates, and financial assistance programs for green home improvements. For example, California's Residential Energy Efficiency Program provides resources and financial assistance for energy-saving upgrades. Websites like EnergySage and the Database of State Incentives for Renewables & Efficiency (DSIRE) can be valuable tools for finding incentives in your area.

Many utility companies also provide rebates and incentives for energy-efficient appliances and home improvements. ENERGY STAR, a program run by the U.S. Environmental Protection Agency (EPA) and the DOE, offers a comprehensive list of energy-efficient products and appliances. You can also find information on utility rebates for ENERGY STAR-certified products on their website.

Lastly, it's essential to stay informed about tax laws and incentives changes. The Inflation Reduction Act of 2022 introduced various tax provisions that impact homeowners and green home renovations.

Five subsidies available through the Inflation Reduction Act include:

1. Enhanced tax credits for electric vehicles: The Inflation Reduction Act has increased the federal tax credit for electric vehicles (EVs), making it more affordable to purchase an EV. These tax credits can be as high as $12,500, depending on the vehicle's price and battery capacity.
2. Extension of the residential renewable energy tax credit: This act (as mentioned earlier) extends the Residential Renewable Energy Tax Credit, allowing homeowners to continue benefiting from tax credits for installing solar panels, wind turbines, and geothermal heat pumps. The credit rate, currently at 26%, will decrease to 22% and is set to expire by 2024.
3. Expansion of the Energy Efficiency Tax Credit: The Inflation Reduction Act expands the Nonbusiness Energy Property Credit, providing more opportunities for homeowners to receive tax credits for energy-saving improvements like insulation, energy-efficient windows, and specific heating and cooling systems.
4. Increased funding for weatherization assistance programs: The act allocates additional funding to the Weatherization Assistance Program, helping low-income households make energy-efficient upgrades and reduce their energy costs. This program provides services like insulation, air sealing, and energy-efficient heating and cooling systems based on the unique needs of each household.
5. Increased funding for state and local energy efficiency programs: The Inflation Reduction Act also provides additional funding for state and local governments to

develop and implement energy efficiency programs. These programs can include tax credits, rebates, and financial assistance for homeowners looking to make green home improvements.

In summary, numerous federal, state, and local incentives are available to support green home renovations. By taking advantage of these programs, homeowners can save money and make eco-friendly upgrades more affordable. Remember to stay informed about changes in incentives and consult with professionals to ensure you make the best decisions for your unique situation.

Impact on home values

Imagine you're a homebuyer. You can pick between a drafty old place with no insulation and ancient toilets that seem to use a hundred gallons per flush, or a shiny, remodeled home with airtight windows and sleek, modern appliances. Which would you choose?

All kidding aside, the data are quite clear. Green updates are popular, increasingly common, and will improve your resale value.

Homeowners love eco-friendly features because they lower utility costs, increase comfort, and reduce environmental impact. A recent report by the National Association of Realtors (NAR) indicates that there has been a sharp increase in the number of homes with green features. According to studies, homes with green features sell faster and at higher prices than their conventional counterparts. Consequently, eco-friendly upgrades can not only save you money on utilities and potentially provide tax incentives, but they can also increase the value of your property.

Here are five green remodels that are most likely to improve property values, along with additional details on their benefits:

1. Solar panels: Installing solar panels can significantly increase your home's value, providing long-term energy savings and reducing dependence on nonrenewable energy sources. Prospective buyers may appreciate solar power's reduced energy costs and environmental impact. Additionally, solar installations can qualify for federal tax credits, further increasing their appeal. Two words of caution here. First, cold, cloudy places don't get much juice from solar panels. And you must be careful with how you finance solar cells. You may reduce the sale price of your home if you encumber it with debt.

2. Energy-efficient windows: Upgrading to ENERGY STAR-certified windows can improve your home's energy efficiency, reduce utility costs, and increase its value. These windows have multiple panes, low-emissivity coatings, and high-quality framing materials that minimize heat transfer and keep your home comfortable year-round. They also help reduce noise pollution and protect your home's interior from UV damage.

3. Insulation and air sealing: Proper insulation can dramatically reduce energy consumption, leading to lower energy bills and a more comfortable living environment. Upgrading attic insulation, sealing gaps and cracks around windows and doors, and insulating walls can all contribute to increased home value. These improvements can make your home more appealing to potential buyers as they demonstrate a commitment to energy efficiency and comfort.

4. Energy-efficient HVAC systems: Replacing outdated heating and cooling systems with energy-efficient models can reduce energy costs and provide a cozier living environment, making your home slam-dunk for buyers. Look for ENERGY STAR-certified HVAC systems, which can save up to 20% on heating and cooling costs compared to standard models. High-efficiency systems may also

qualify for tax credits and rebates, increasing their appeal and your sale price.

5. Water-saving fixtures: Installing water-efficient fixtures, such as low-flow faucets, showerheads, and toilets, can help conserve water and reduce utility costs. In addition to saving money on water bills, water-efficient fixtures can reduce the strain on local water resources and contribute to a more sustainable living environment. These upgrades are no-brainers in parched areas with high water costs.

Projected savings from Energy Star, solar, dual-pane windows, and water-saving fixtures

Here's a more detailed look at the potential savings associated with Energy Star appliances, solar panels, dual-pane windows, and water-saving fixtures:

1. Energy Star appliances: ENERGY STAR certified machines use 10-50% less energy than standard models. Replacing your old appliances with ENERGY STAR-certified models can save you hundreds of dollars in energy costs over their lifetimes. These savings can vary based on regional energy costs, usage patterns, and your chosen appliances. For example, an ENERGY STAR-certified refrigerator can save up to $300 over its lifetime compared to a non-certified model, while an ENERGY STAR-certified clothes washer can save up to $380. Additionally, some utility companies offer rebates for purchasing ENERGY STAR-certified appliances, further increasing the potential savings (see above).

2. Solar panels: Solar panels can substantially reduce or even eliminate your electricity bill, depending on the size of the system and the amount of sunlight your home receives. The average homeowner with a solar installation can save between $10,000 and $30,000 over the system's 20- to 25-year lifespan, depending on their location, system size, and

local electricity rates. Homeowners in sunnier regions like the Southwest can expect tremendous savings, while those in cloudier areas like the Pacific Northwest will see little value. Additionally, the federal solar tax credit allows you to deduct 26% of the cost of your solar installation from your federal taxes, further increasing the financial benefits. The good news is that this technology seems to improve daily. Get ready to kiss your coal-powered lights goodbye.

3. Dual-pane windows: Replacing single-pane windows with energy-efficient dual-pane windows can save you an estimated $126-$465 per year on energy costs, depending on your climate and the type of windows you choose. Dual-pane windows, especially those with low-emissivity (Low-E) coatings, are designed to minimize heat transfer, reducing the amount of heat that enters your home in the summer and exits in the winter. This can help you maintain a comfortable indoor temperature while reducing reliance on heating and cooling systems. The potential savings from dual-pane windows will be greater in regions with more extreme temperatures, as homeowners typically spend more on heating and cooling.

4. Water-saving fixtures: Installing water-efficient fixtures, such as low-flow faucets, showerheads, and toilets, can help conserve water and reduce utility costs. For example, replacing an older toilet with a WaterSense-labeled high-efficiency toilet can save the average family nearly 13,000 gallons of water per year, resulting in annual water savings of more than $110. For reference, that's almost enough water to fill a home swimming pool! Similarly, replacing a standard showerhead with a WaterSense-labeled model can save an average of 2,700 gallons per year, resulting in annual water savings of over $70. These savings can be even more significant in areas with water scarcity or high water costs. In addition to saving money on water bills, water-efficient

fixtures can reduce the strain on local water resources and contribute to a more sustainable living environment.

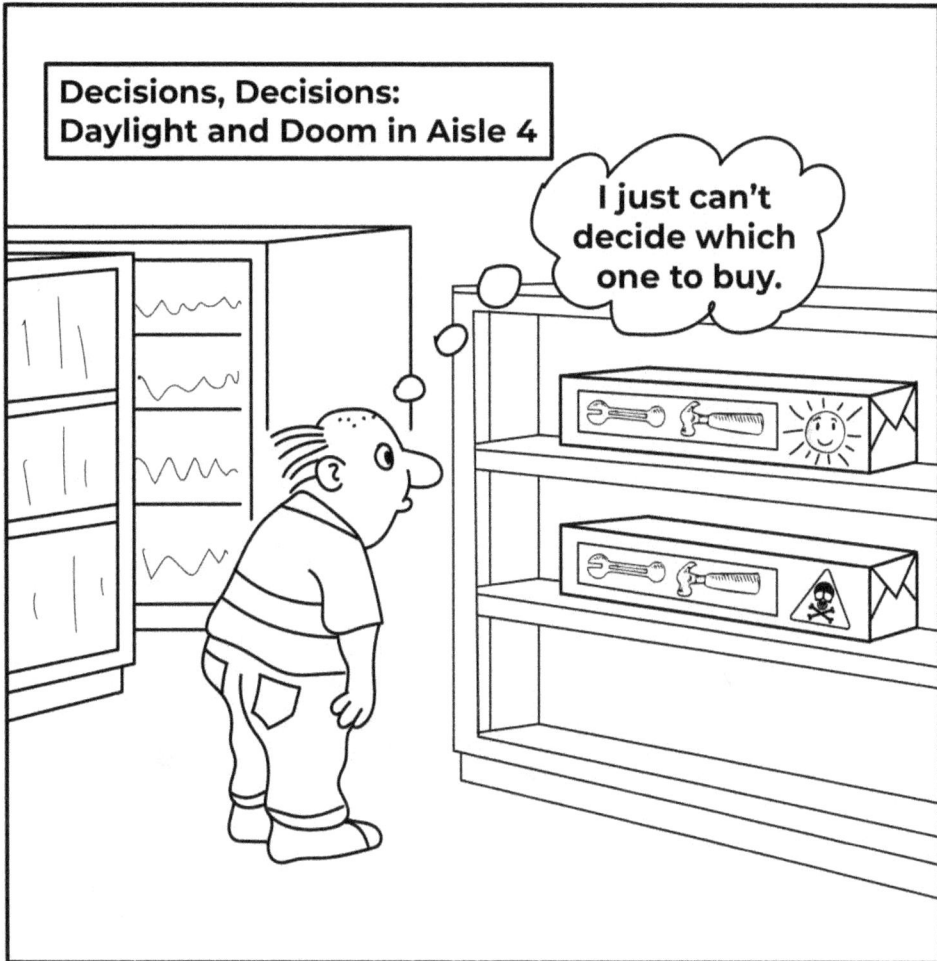

Choosing which remodels have the greatest bang for your buck is all about location. Utility costs, climate, and individual usage patterns should drive your decisions. If you're in a sunny and dry area, get the water-saving stuff and consider solar. If you're in the cold northeast, you really can't have too much insulation. And we can all do our part with energy-saving appliances. Your buyers and the planet will love you for it.

Interview: Ron Watson

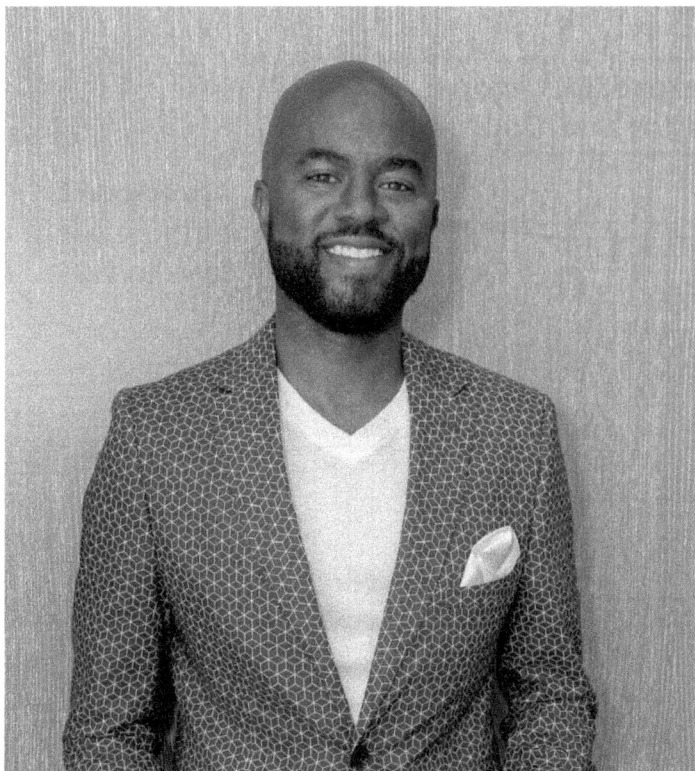

Rod Watson is a premier agent in California's thriving Los Angeles and San Diego luxury real estate markets. With a remarkable 17-year career in the industry that began with his first home purchase in 2005, Watson has carved out a unique niche as an agent to the stars. His rich knowledge of eco-friendly renovations and innate ability to anticipate high-net-worth buyers' expectations have set him apart in sustainable luxury living.

Watson's athletic background instilled in him the values of discipline and hard work. He translated these qualities from the basketball court into real estate, tailoring his services to cater specifically to professional athletes and entertainers, a clientele he understands on a personal and cultural level. His sensitivity to their elite lifestyle needs and his astute awareness of sustainable trends enables him to offer guidance on renovating properties to maximize their market value and appeal.

As part of his comprehensive service, Watson often provides advice on pre-sale renovations. These remodels, from minor cosmetic updates to major overhauls of kitchens and bathrooms, tap into current trends and affluent buyer preferences. He said millennials and other young buyers often seek "turn-key" homes, ready for immediate occupancy without additional updates. This strategy and a quick turnaround time of 60-90 days can significantly enhance property values and accelerate sales.

Watson's approach to aesthetics combines functionality with style. He often suggests wood flooring, quartz countertops, and light, neutral paint colors to give homes a fresh, contemporary feel. Recessed lighting is another commonly recommended feature, bringing a modern touch to any space.

However, Watson's expertise extends beyond cosmetic upgrades. He is a leader in integrating eco-friendly and energy-efficient features, which are increasingly in demand among luxury buyers. With California's solar mandate requiring all new single-family homes built post-2020 to be equipped with rooftop solar photovoltaic systems, Watson understands the importance of such sustainable upgrades.

Incorporating double-pane windows, solar panels, smart home technology, tankless hot water heaters, and energy-efficient appliances into his renovations, Watson ensures these homes are up to par with his state's environmental expectations. His properties often include EV chargers, dual-zone thermostats, and even whole-home automation systems, which are operable from an iPad and reflect the high-end market's desire for cutting-edge technology.

Beyond the walls of the home, Watson's eco-friendly philosophy continues. He proposes beautiful, sustainable gardens featuring low-maintenance, water-efficient plants like succulents and palm trees. Water-conserving drip irrigation systems are a must. These landscape designs adhere to the West's water restrictions while adding a touch of serene beauty to his properties.

Watson's clientele is diverse. While some ultra-luxury buyers seek expansive homes of 5,000-15,000 square feet with multi-generation suites, he has noticed a growing trend towards smaller, easy-to-maintain spaces among experienced buyers without children.

Rod Watson is a Texas Native and former Athlete setting an incomparable standard among his peers in Real Estate. Rod has achieved esteemed recognition throughout Southern California for his high-net-worth clientele and complimentary services. Since 2008, Rod has amassed more than $200+ million in sales volume, $24.9 million of which was in 2022 alone. Specializing in serving athletes, entertainment professionals, investors, and developers, Rod flexes industry prestige that has garnered the trust of so many notable clientele and attracted the attention of several major publications. He has frequently contributed to the San Diego Business Journal and the Los Angeles Business Journal, the San Diego Union-Tribune, Forbes, The Real Deal magazine, ESPN, Mansion Global, and the Los Angeles Times.

Growing up in Texas as a hybrid city-country boy, Rod played college basketball before playing professionally in Brazil and coaching the sport while earning his master's degree in counseling and business management at Point Loma Nazarene University. That experience gave him the leadership, instincts, and problem-solving skills inherent in athletes and the ability not only to advise clients about buying and selling real estate but also about building wealth, never forgetting that each transaction is profoundly affecting. Rod further boosts his niche value with his cultural perspective, financial background, and personal real estate investment experience, and so he understands firsthand the importance of discretion. He also holds Certified Luxury Home

Marketing Specialist and Short Sales and Foreclosure Resource designations and Million Dollar Guild recognition.

Inspired to launch a real estate career to live life on his terms and create generational wealth for his family, Rod is passionate about helping his clients do the same. Through unparalleled value and resourcefulness, Rod simultaneously strives to build his name, business, and network and leave a legacy for his daughters.

Contact Information

Interested in learning more about California's luxury real estate market? You can contact Rod at rod@distinctconciergere.com *or give him a call at 323-615-1963.*

CHAPTER 16

Case Studies:

Three Green Home Remodels

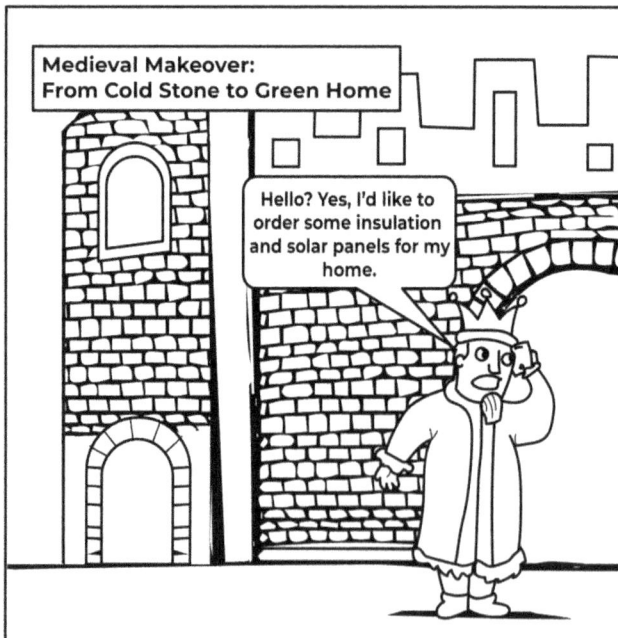

Remodel 1: $15,000 Renovation for a Mid-Century House in Los Angeles, CA

The Ramirez family, residents of sunny Hollywood, recently embarked on a green home remodel journey for their mid-century house. Their home was made famous in 1994 as the site of a campy TV drama, so they wanted to preserve the house's aesthetics. With a budget of $15,000, their main goal was to increase the energy efficiency of their home while minimizing their carbon footprint and ultimately reducing their utility bills.

They researched eco-friendly home improvements that would match their minimalist architecture and found various ways to make their home greener while staying within budget. They began with Mid-century style magazines Dwell and Atomic Ranch to find innovative ways to draw in natural light and brighten colors so they wouldn't need as much artificial lighting. Then they turned to resources like the California Green Building Standards (CalGreen) and CalRecycle to learn about sustainable building practices and state incentives.

Solar Panels

The Ramirez family decided to invest in solar panels to generate clean, renewable energy. After investigating, they discovered California is one of the best states for solar power, thanks to its abundant sunshine and incentives. They contacted a local solar installation company that helped them design a 3-kilowatt system tailored to their home's energy needs and roof orientation. Thankfully, they could hide the panels to make them nearly invisible from the front of the house.

The total cost for the solar system, including installation, was $7,500. This investment would help them save on utility bills while reducing their reliance on fossil fuels.

Energy-Efficient Appliances

To further improve their home's energy efficiency, the Ramirez family upgraded their appliances to Energy Star-certified models. They replaced their old refrigerator, washing machine, and dishwasher with energy-efficient counterparts, spending $4,000 on these upgrades. By doing so, they would save energy and reduce their water consumption, leading to lower utility bills. Plus, they looked great in their kitchen!

Drought-Tolerant Landscaping and Hardscaping

Living in sunny Los Angeles, the Ramirez family recognized the importance of water conservation. They decided to transform their landscaping by incorporating drought-tolerant plants and installing a drip irrigation system. They carefully selected native plants such as California lilacs, manzanitas, and succulents that require minimal water and maintenance. These plants save water and attract local wildlife like birds and butterflies, creating a vibrant ecosystem in their yard.

To further conserve water, they replaced a portion of their lawn with permeable pavers and decomposed granite, reducing the amount of turf that needed regular watering. They also added a few cactuses, which they enjoyed more than their old lawn.

They also incorporated a rainwater harvesting system, including a rain barrel, to collect and store rainwater for their garden. The total cost for their eco-friendly landscaping and hardscaping project was around $3,500.

Rebates and Incentives

The Ramirez family applied for various rebates and incentives to help with the cost of their green remodels. They were eligible for the California Solar Initiative (CSI) rebates, which provide financial incentives for solar energy systems. They also took advantage of the federal solar tax credit, which allows homeowners to claim up to 26% of the cost of their solar installation on their taxes.

Moreover, they applied for the Inflation Reduction Act Residential Energy Rebate Programs in California, which offers rebates on energy-efficient appliances. These subsidies helped them offset the cost of their appliance upgrades and made their updates more affordable.

Overall, the Ramirez family completed their $15,000 green remodel, improving their home's energy efficiency and reducing environmental impact. They are now enjoying a more comfortable home with lower utility bills while contributing to a greener future. Their drought-tolerant landscaping and solar panels serve as inspiring examples for their neighbors and community, showcasing the benefits of sustainable living. Even better, they're now ready next time a famous movie producer comes knocking on their door!

Remodel 2: $15,000 Green Update for a 100-Year-Old Townhouse in Boston, MA

The O'Malley family, living in a historic 100-year-old townhouse in Boston, was determined to make their home more energy-efficient and eco-friendly. With a budget of $15,000, they aimed to improve the comfort of their home during the cold Boston winters, address the unique challenges of their townhouse, and preserve its historic charm.

The O'Malleys started by researching various green home improvement projects and exploring resources like Mass Save, Mass.gov, and Boston.gov to learn about sustainable options and available incentives in Massachusetts.

Window and Insulation Upgrade

To better protect their home from the harsh Boston winters and improve energy efficiency, the O'Malleys decided to upgrade their windows and insulation. They replaced their single-pane windows with double-pane, energy-efficient models, which would help keep their home warmer during the winter and cooler in the summer. The total cost for window replacements was around $4,000.

Their new windows added light and matched the neighborhood's upscale architecture.

They added insulation to their attic, walls, and basement. Additional insulation reduces drafts, improves comfort, and lowers heating bills. They chose a combination of spray foam and cellulose insulation made from eco-friendly materials to provide optimal thermal performance. The insulation project cost approximately $6,000.

Air Sealing and Energy Audit

Given the age of their townhouse, the O'Malleys wanted to address potential air leaks that could affect their home's energy efficiency. They scheduled an energy audit with a local contractor, who assessed their home for air leaks and energy-saving opportunities. After the audit, the contractor recommended air sealing around windows, doors, and other gaps to prevent drafts and heat loss. The energy audit and air sealing measures cost around $1,500.

High-Efficiency Heating System

Considering their townhouse's unique layout and heating requirements, the O'Malleys invested in a new heating system. They chose a modern, energy-efficient boiler to provide consistent and comfortable heat while reducing energy consumption. The state-of-the-art boiler would lower their carbon footprint and save on heating costs. The cost for the heater, including installation, was around $3,500.

Rebates and Incentives

To help offset the costs of their green home renovations, the O'Malleys applied for various rebates and incentives. They participated in the Mass Save program, which offers no-cost home energy assessments and financial incentives for energy-efficient upgrades. Through the program, they received rebates for their window replacements, insulation upgrades, and high-efficiency heating system.

They also took advantage of the Residential Energy Property Tax Credit. This federal program allows homeowners to claim up to 10% of the cost of eligible energy-efficient improvements, including windows and insulation.

The O'Malleys were thrilled with their $15,000 green update for their 100-year-old Boston townhouse by making these eco-friendly improvements. Since all of the renovations were in the interior of their home (except the windows), they remained true to their neighborhood's historic character. They addressed the unique challenges of their historic home and enhanced its energy efficiency, ensuring a comfortable and environmentally friendly living space for years to come.

Remodel 3: $60,000 Overhaul for a Suburban House in Atlanta, GA

In leafy Atlanta, the Johnson family was eager to make substantial eco-friendly changes to their suburban house. With a generous budget of $60,000, they aimed to improve their home's energy efficiency, reduce its environmental impact, and create a healthier living space for their family. They started by researching various green remodeling projects and consulting resources like their home warranty and utility companies to learn about sustainable options and available incentives in Georgia.

Geothermal Heating and Cooling System

The Johnsons wanted to go big, so they took the plunge and scored a geothermal heating and cooling system. As early adopters, they were excited by this technology's potential for long-term energy savings and environmental benefits. After thorough research, they selected a geothermal heat pump that uses the earth's stable underground temperature to provide efficient heating and cooling. The installation cost was $20,000, but they estimated the system would slash their energy bills by up to 60% in the long run.

Solar Water Heater

In addition to the geothermal system, the Johnsons installed a solar water heater. This system would harness the sun's power to heat their water, reducing their reliance on nonrenewable energy sources. They spent $4,000 on the solar water heater, which could cut their water heating costs by up to 80%.

Low VOC Paint and Materials

Not everything is pricy! The Johnson family worried about the indoor air quality of their home since they had young children. They decided to repaint the interior of their house using low VOC (volatile organic compound) paints, which emit fewer harmful chemicals and have less impact on indoor air quality. In addition, they replaced their old carpet with eco-friendly flooring made from sustainable materials like bamboo and cork. The cost of the painting and flooring projects was around $8,000.

Kitchen Remodel with Energy-Efficient Appliances and Sustainable Materials

Next, the Johnsons refreshed their kitchen. They replaced their old appliances with Energy Star-certified models, including a new refrigerator, dishwasher, and range. The family also opted for sustainable materials in their kitchen renovation, such as recycled glass countertops and sustainably harvested wood for their cabinetry. Using these eco-friendly materials reduced their home's environmental impact and created a healthier living space. The total cost of the kitchen remodels was $25,000.

Rainwater Harvesting System and Native Plant Landscaping

Finally, the Johnsons rigged a rainwater harvesting system to collect and store rainwater for their garden. They installed a 500-gallon rain barrel and connected it to their home's gutter system. This rainwater is perfect for watering their plants, reducing their reliance on municipal water supplies.

To complement their rainwater harvesting system, the Johnsons redesigned their landscaping using native plants that thrive in Georgia's climate. These plants require less water and maintenance, making them ideal for the family's eco-friendly goals. They also incorporated a drip irrigation system to water their plants while conserving water efficiently. Plus, it's a huge time-saver! The rainwater harvesting system and landscaping changes cost around $3,000.

Rebates and Incentives

The Johnson family took advantage of several rebates and incentives to offset the cost of their green home renovations. They applied for federal tax credits for geothermal heating and cooling systems, which allowed them to claim up to 26% of the cost of their geothermal system on their taxes. They also claimed a federal tax credit for their solar water heater, which covered 26% of its price.

Additionally, they researched and applied for local Atlanta Gas & Light rebates, which provided incentives for energy-efficient appliance upgrades and home improvements. They also took advantage of Georgia's Green Energy Program, which offered tax credits for renewable energy systems, including solar water heaters.

Overall, the Johnson family completed their $60,000 green home renovation, incorporating a variety of sustainable improvements that significantly increased their home's energy efficiency and reduced its environmental impact. Their investment in a geothermal heating and cooling system, solar water heater, eco-friendly kitchen remodel, low VOC paint, sustainable flooring, rainwater harvesting system, and native plant landscaping has transformed their suburban house into a healthier and more sustainable living space.

Not only did the Johnsons make their home more comfortable and environmentally friendly, but they also inspired their neighbors and community to consider eco-friendly home improvements. A local design magazine featured their high-powered home on the cover!

Conclusion

Imagine finding yourself transported back in time, standing on London's iconic river embankment in 1957. You're surrounded by the city's historical grandeur with the stately Big Ben in the distance. Yet, your senses are overwhelmed by the sight and stench of the River Thames, which bears little resemblance to the vibrant waterway that once coursed through the heart of this great city.

For centuries, the Thames had been the lifeblood of London. King Henry VIII would embark on royal processions up and down the river, and in May 1533, Anne Boleyn traveled along it to her crowning as Queen. The river was witness to both grand celebrations and solemn occasions. It was the heart of trade, a thoroughfare of culture, and the backdrop to London's transformation from a Roman outpost to an imperial metropolis.

But the river, once integral to life and livelihoods, had transformed over time into a swirling cesspool. The state of the River Thames was so perilous in the 1950s that tumbling into its waters meant an immediate trip to the hospital to pump your stomach, given the river was teeming with raw sewage. A cocktail of industrial waste and household trash replaced its once-clean waters. Instead of mirroring the proud face of Big Ben, the river's surface was now a canvas for a grim tableau of pollution. The smell was overwhelming—an unholy mix of rot, decay, and chemical tang that permeated everything it touched.

Fast forward to the present day, at the start of the 21st century, and the Thames has undergone a rebirth. The Thames did not transform from an environmental disaster to a beacon of hope through luck. Instead, it was the result of deliberate and sustained human effort.

The catalysts for the formation in the late 20th century were civic activism, government leadership, and the Thames Water Authority.

They rose like a phoenix to save the river. One of their critical initiatives was the construction of new sewage treatment plants. Using advanced processes such as activated sludge and aerated biological filters, these facilities removed harmful pollutants before they could reach the river.

But the cleanup wasn't just about cutting off the river's pollution sources. The river itself needed healing. Officials installed air bubblers across the length of the Thames. These devices pumped much-needed oxygen into the water, fostering an environment where aquatic life could survive and eventually thrive.

Over time, the river began to regain its vigor. Invertebrates returned, their presence attracting fish and birds. The Thames is now home to over 125 fish species. Seals and even dolphins started splashing around in its waters. The reflection of Big Ben once again graces the river's surface, a sight that seemed unimaginable a few decades ago.

The transformation of the Thames from a neglected wasteland to a revitalized ecosystem is a powerful testament to what is possible when society commits to environmental stewardship. The story of the Thames is an embodiment of the belief that it is never too late to make a difference. It's a shining example of how history and progress can coexist, and how we can preserve our past while ensuring a sustainable future.

Emerging from the River Thames epic transformation tale, we're confronted by a remarkable truth. Here's the river, once the lifeblood of an empire, then an open sewer, and now, a symbol of environmental rejuvenation. This turnabout reveals a profound intersection between the health of our environment and our well-being.

Consider the River Thames' journey. Its pollution was not merely an ecological disaster; it posed significant health risks to London's residents and their pets. As the river recovered, so did the people and animals that depended on it. Cleaner water meant fewer pollutants in the air and soil, which translated into fewer health issues for humans and animals alike. When we enhance the environment's health, we inevitably improve our health and that of our pets.

In July 2023, I had the privilege of witnessing the River Thames' transformation firsthand. Its renaissance left me speechless. I wholeheartedly salute the British people for their unyielding efforts to restore this river to its splendid beauty.

Now, let's shift this idea from the grand scale of a city's river to the intimate spaces of our homes. We often view environmental sustainability as a concept outside our front doors—an issue for industries, governments, and cities to tackle. However, an equally potent site of transformation exists much closer than you might think. Your living room. Your kitchen. Your backyard.

Sustainability starts at home.

But how does one imbue a house with sustainability? It's easier than it sounds. Take, for instance, the wood you might use for your decking or the new bookshelf you're planning. Sustainable woods, such as bamboo or reclaimed timber, are environmentally friendly, incredibly durable, and look great.

Likewise, your choice of paints can make a difference. Traditional paints often contain Volatile Organic Compounds (VOCs), contributing to air pollution and can cause various health issues. By choosing low or zero-VOC versions, you cleanse the atmosphere within and outside your home.

Even everyday cleaning can be an act of environmental stewardship. Conventional cleaning products are often tested on animals and loaded with harmful chemicals. On the other hand, natural household cleaners—many made from everyday pantry items like vinegar, baking soda, and lemon—are affordable and just as effective. They're gentler on the environment and safer for you and your pets.

Let's appreciate the power of energy efficiency. Appliances guzzle energy, but they don't have to. Energy-efficient appliances, from refrigerators to washing machines, reduce the strain on our planet's resources while lowering utility bills. Efficient HVAC systems will save you a bundle.

And the environmental potential of our homes doesn't end at the backdoor. Better landscape design can minimize water usage, promote local biodiversity, and even improve the energy efficiency of your house. For example, strategically planting trees for shade can reduce the need for air conditioning in the summer.

Our homes are not just places to live; they're places where we can make a difference. Every sustainable choice will help preserve our shared planet and give our kids and pets the nurturing environment they need to thrive.

The River Thames did not clean itself. It was a conscious decision by a determined society. Similarly, our homes will not magically become sustainable. It requires deliberate actions by each of us, and it's a journey that can start today.

Look around your home. Every object, every appliance, and every square foot is an opportunity to contribute to a greener world. And if the transformation of the Thames teaches us anything it is that change is possible. Everything we do makes a difference. Remember, sustainability starts at home. Because, in the end, the health of the planet rests on our choices.

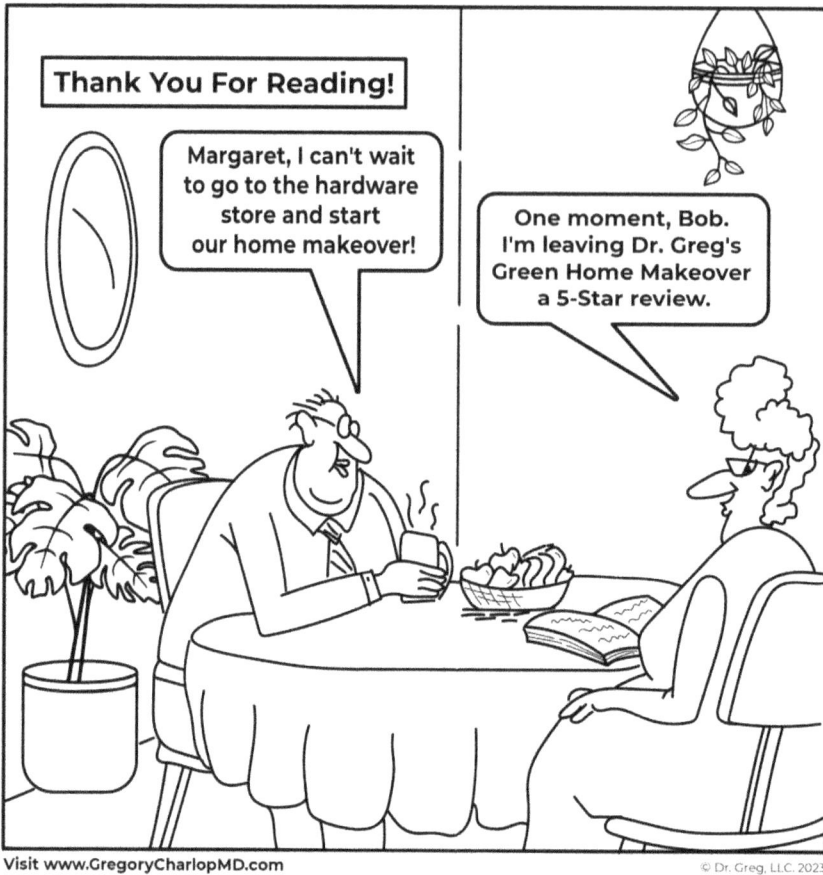

If you found this book helpful, please share it with a friend and write an honest, 5-star review online. And if you have any questions or would like to explore the possibility of my team visiting your home or office in person or by video for a custom makeover, feel free to reach out to me on LinkedIn or my website, www.GregoryCharlopMD.com.

Take care, and together we can protect the planet for the next generation!

Gregory Charlop, MD

www.ingramcontent.com/pod-product-compliance
Lightning Source LLC
Chambersburg PA
CBHW052110020426

42335CB00021B/2696